MW00932393

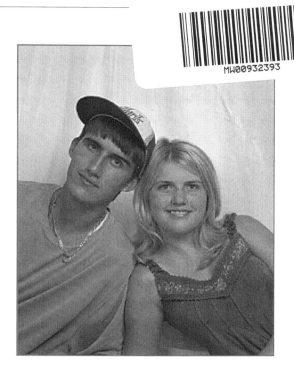

Tom and his sister
Amanda 2007

Brian O – Wow. Amazing and inspirational story Randy. Your open and honest record of your journey with Tom will I'm sure give hope and courage to anyone who is struggling to deal with the challenges life throws at us.

Jan G – I barely breathed until the last sentence. Congratulations on the story and the life

Leonardo B- It takes a real Man to have the courage to write down this story. As we struggle we some medical issues in our family, I look at the file I´ve just downloaded with a strange mix of reverence and fear. I always pray for all of you.

Michelle – I felt like I was there, crying, laughing and gasping for air. My prayers go out to Tom and Randy, along with my thanks for sharing this story of hope.

Introduction

Sometimes you hold onto a strand of light, because you think that is all you have, all you can hope for. Then you look back and find you have been hugging the sun.

This is the story of my son Tom and me, and of a remarkable journey down a path that no parent ever wants to walk, and that no kid should have to endure. It's also the beginning of the story of Tom, an amazing individual. Tom endured a total of 14 surgeries over 13 years. Three times, he has had a major resection, inflicting severe trauma to his brain. Three times he has had to teach himself to walk again. With each trauma of surgery came waves of pain, heavy and addictive pain medications, and resistance to those medications. This is the story of a young boy looking for the strength to battle through extreme circumstances to become a man.

This is my story too--the story of a father of two, a beautiful young girl, and an energetic boy with a magnetic personality and smile. It's a story about missing clues and changing my mind about what I thought I knew, what I thought was right. It's a story about the friends and the people I love. Some I have known since I was young, some are new, and many have come and gone, but all have left a dramatic impression as they supported me in my fight to support my son.

My family has been amazing. Despite difficult challenges of their own, they have not hesitated in their support or love for Tom and me. I have never questioned whether they would be there when we needed them. Until now, as I am writing this, it never even occurred to me that they had an option, or could have ever thought of giving anything less.

Then there is Amanda, "Bug", my daughter. She has also been a victim of the tumor. Early in her life we were separated, and this, combined with my urgent need to focus on Tom's care, gave us little time together. I was absent for some of the most important times of her life, and yet she has grown to become a beautiful and caring young woman. As I write, she is focused on her studies to become a nurse, and I have no doubt that she will be wonderful at her chosen occupation.

There are many incredible events in this story. Unique opportunities arose, all of which Tom paid for in illness and pain. Much of my growth over the years, as well as my pain, came about because he suffered. I met remarkable people and experienced extraordinary events, and I feel guilty. Why should I benefit as my kids suffer? Though I greatly value these people and experiences, the circumstances surrounding them continue to weigh heavily on my soul. And yet, despite all of this, I can't help but feel that we are fortunate.

In writing this, I know that there will be important people, doctors, friends, and events that I will miss. Others may have views that are different from what I remember and feel, but this is my story, and I share it for those that may find strength and hope in it. I share this story to show the strength in Tom, and the strength he has given me. I share this to say thanks to my family and friends. And I share this for me, so that I may be thankful and not forget.

Chapter 1 - Into the Dark, the First Days

My son started thrashing around in his sleeping bag at midnight on August 16th, 2000. I immediately felt startled and concerned. I had never seen my son have a seizure before, but I knew what it was, and knew that it would likely subside quickly, as it did. I got him up and walked around. He was confused, dazed, and not feeling well. A bit unsteady on his feet, but I expected that. He did not seem to be in immediate danger, so I laid my 12-year-old son back in his sleeping bag, and watched him sleep for the rest of the night. We were at a family reunion with my in-laws, camping a few miles outside Richfield, Utah. Beth's family lived in Richfield and her sister had just returned after being gone on a Mission for the Mormon Church for 18 months. Beth, her other two sisters, her two brothers and parents were all there to celebrate the return.

The next morning I called his doctor in Oregon, then took him to the small hospital in Richfield for an examination. Tom's stepmother, Beth, and Beth's mother Cathy rode with us. I was extremely alarmed at Tom's appearance. His eyes we glazed, and he was very sedate. Not normal for a kid some thought had ADHD.

In the hospital the doctor did an examination, then left to make a quick call. He came back and we took my son into a room for a CAT scan. I stood next to him as his head and upper body made the trip through the large circular apparatus. He did really well, lying there calm and still with his long thin body stretched out on the narrow table. It only took a couple of minutes, then the technician led me out the door and directly into the room with monitors. There were three men in their late forties, standing around the screen. When one of them spoke, a doctor, my world changed forever. I can still hear the words today, as clearly as at that moment.

"Mr. Dahl, there is no easy way to tell you this. You son has a large brain tumor and he is in trouble. We have spoken to the doctors at Children's hospital, and they recommend you get him there as quickly as possible."

I was shocked; I didn't know how to react. There is a hospital in Portland, closer to where we live, called Doernbecher's. It is supposed to be a great children's hospital, should we go there? I asked the question and the doctors recommended that we go to Primary Children's Hospital in Salt Lake City as quickly as we could.

I grabbed Tom, Beth, and Cathy, and we left. The campsite was on the way, so we could drop Cathy off there, pick up our daughter, and then leave all our gear, clothes and food. People have odd thoughts at times of pressure. Cathy said she wanted to stop and get buttermilk for breakfast. Why was she focusing on that? I could barely drive or think. Tom was in the seat next to me, and his head ached. He had been having headaches for some time, but the doctors said they were just growing pains, stress. Now he was hurting and quiet. We raced to the campsite. When we arrived, Cathy jumped out and we packed our daughter Amanda and our dog Charlie into our red 95 Jimmy and took off.

I don't remember much of the drive, but I remember the emotions. Even today it is extremely difficult to think about. The tears start, the panic builds, and my body feels weak and drained. What I do remember are the words Tom said. "Dad, it's OK, I am not afraid to die". I tried to be strong, assure him that everything would be ok. But I could not talk much. I had to concentrate on driving and not breaking down in a wave of panic.

When we got to the emergency door of Children's Hospital in Salt Lake City, they were waiting for us. Someone asked why we had not been on a Life Flight. The doctor had left the room to coordinate the flight. I did not know what he was doing, no one mentioned an emergency flight to Salt Lake City, but I did feel the urgency of time so I just scooped up Tom and headed for Children's without waiting.

Within minutes, we were in a room and the doctors and staff were taking vital signs and hooking Tom to IVs. Inside of 15 minutes, Tom was sedated and Dr. Walker had drilled a small hole in his skull to relieve the pressure. Tom's tumor had closed off the ventricles that drain excess fluid from the brain, and the pressure had mounted, causing the headaches and seizure he had experienced. It had caused enough damage that Dr. Walker told us Tom would never have survived the trip back to Oregon.

Twenty minutes later, Tom came out of sedation, and was talking and feeling better. He is a kid that loves to talk--always has. He is clear and and can go on for hours. His reasoning can be off, but he can go on for hours. "What is a Zebra? 26 sizes larger than an A bra." He would tell that joke no fewer than 20 times over the next two weeks to every nurse, doctor, orderly and visitor.

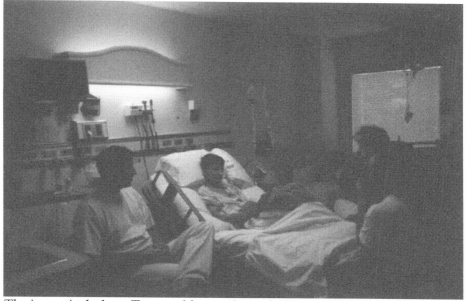

The image is dark, as Tom could not tolerate light or a flash without extreme pain. In the picture is Tom, Randy, Beth and a videographer who is making a video to support the Ronald McDonald House fund raising efforts.

Over the next hour, the Children's doctors performed several tests on Tom, an MRI to get better images of the tumor, blood tests, reflex tests, and many that I am, and will probably never be, aware of. During one such test, a light was shone directly into his eye to look at the nerves in the back of the eyeball. The eye is the only place that you can look directly at nerves. As Children's is a teaching hospital, Dr. Walker had several residents, students, and nurses come look at the nerves in the back of his eye. They kept coming until Tom asked them to stop, indicating that it was causing him discomfort. Dr. Walker explained that the pressure in Tom's brain caused the nerves in his eye to "stick out". It was a tell-tale sign of the pressure, and presented a fairly unique teaching opportunity. About an hour after we arrived at Children's hospital, Dr. Walker came out to speak to Beth and me. He told us that the tumor was large and needed to be removed immediately. It was on the left cerebellum which is the part of the brain that controls speaking and coordination. He would not know for sure until after the surgery and a biopsy, but Dr. Walker suspected that the tumor was malignant, and either had or would spread, based on its growth pattern and size. Tom was in deep trouble. Dr. Walker scheduled emergency surgery for the next day at 6:00 AM. We were told that after the surgery Tom might not be able to walk or talk, but would need intense therapy.

That night Pam, Tom's biological mother, came to the hospital from Sandy, Utah. My parents, my sister, her husband, and one of her sons, Jacob, drove in from Sandy, Oregon. Tom's Stepmother Beth, Amanda and I were there. We were all there for Tom, to support him, pray for him and hope for him. Tom asked about me and my job.

"Dad, you can go back if you need to work. Won't you get fired if you are here with me, instead of working?" He told me he would be OK. He wasn't afraid to die, but he did not want to hurt. I told him that we walked into the hospital together, and we would walk out together--nothing would stop that.

The next morning, August 17, 2000, Doctor Marion Walker began a twelve and a half hour surgery to remove a tumor the size of a large peach from Tom's brain. This was the beginning of a personal darkness that I cannot explain. For Tom, it was the beginning of a thirteen year period of pain and struggle--of challenges that shaped his young life and still confront him today. It was a time of intense emotions that both bonded and tore apart. A time where support was needed and love flowed.

Waiting

My parents, Ray and Charlotte, my sister Michele, her husband Steve, and her youngest son Jacob arrived early on the morning of the 17th. They took turns coming in to see Tom, expressing concern the best way they could and sharing tears and love. Pam was there at the hospital and did the best she could as well. What could we do?

I held Tom's hand while they prepared him for surgery. Again, not everyone could come in at once, so Beth, his sister, my parents, and his mom all came in and out. The doctors, nurses and staff were kind and did their best to make us all comfortable, while dedicating all attention possible to Tom and his plight. Dr. Walker came and explained again what was happening and the possible side effects, including loss of speech, the ability to walk, and pain. We were also reminded that Tom's life was in danger and this surgery carried a great risk of death. He did not know what he would find, but would do his best to remove the tumor and leave Tom whole.

Beth intercepted anyone that had administrative issues for us to deal with. She found the places to sit, clean up, eat, and pray. She handled the admission papers, consent forms, address verifications and insurance issues. The paperwork is amazing. We knew we were going to be there for some time, so she found everyone a place to stay. She contacted the Ronald McDonald house and grabbed a room there. So many things that had to be done, but I did not have the sense of mind to accomplish any of it.

Tom was taken into surgery and the waiting began. A darkness surrounded me then that I have trouble explaining, and even now, there is a part of it in my soul. I have always been a planner, a visionary, a person that looks to the future. I set goals, and always have a vision of where I want to be, how I want to look, and who I want to be with. I continually set goals for the day, week, month and year. I evaluate and re-evaluate. I had a wife and family that I loved, supported and who supported me. But during this time, I could not see or feel any of it. I could not imagine one second ahead of the moment we were in. It took every effort just to complete tasks like breathing, watching the seconds on the clock, or talking. I did not know if it was day or night, and I don't think I cared. It took all my life energy to think of Tom.

Can you play?

It was 5:30 am when the phone woke me up. It was ringing at the side of my bed, the old style ring, extra loud. The first thing I did was to try and ignore it--they can leave a message. Who the hell would be calling me at 5:30 am on a Saturday? The sun was just starting to come up, lighting the room and warming the house. It was summer and it was going to be a hot one.

Our house was a split entry home in Pleasant Grove, Utah. The home sat on a hill, about a tenth of the way up, where the houses ended and the grass and rock took over. If you continued to climb you would reach a large "G" made by placing rocks in formation and then painting them white. This is very common for the areas around Utah as a show of community spirit for schools and towns.

The house was situated on a corner of the narrow suburban street, with neighbors on two sides and the mountain rising up behind the house to the east. The yard was fenced, with a large old apricot tree in the back. It was a great place to live, but that damn phone started ringing again.

Normally I would have been out of the house on a weekend like this, headed up the canyon, past Sundance Ski Resort, and up to Deer Creek Reservoir, to do some water-skiing, but today I was sleeping in. Well, I would be sleeping in if that fool on the phone would quit calling. It had been a long week, I was tired, and this was irritating. Finally the phone stopped ringing, and then the knocks came.

Someone was knocking on the door, loudly. I got out of bed and fumbled to get my jeans on and walked to the stairs with squinty eyes, and black hair sticking up forming some weird type of semi-mohawk. I was not wearing a shirt or shoes; whoever was at the door would have to deal with me the way I was.

At the bottom of the stairs I noticed a chair, right up against the door. That was really odd--why did Pam put a chair against the door? She wasn't trying to lock anyone out and there was no one else here, except Tom, and he was only four.

I was tired. I was grumpy. I moved the chair and opened the door. "It better not be any kind of door to door sales" was the thought that ran through my mind. And what about missionaries? No, they are not that stupid, besides, they would be sleeping too. Then, as I opened the door I saw them. My next door neighbor and Tom, my four year old son that, last I knew, was in bed.

Tom was full of life and energy, and he did not have time to waste waiting for all the big people to finally get up. There was sunshine, it was warm, and he wanted to play. Now he was holding hands with the neighbor and sporting an enormous smile. He was almost always smiling, but when he knew he was going to be in trouble, the smile doubled in size. So Tom and his smile had crawled out of bed sometime around 5:00 am, grabbed a chair to climb on, taken it down the stairs and used it as a ladder so he could reach the door locks and escape the house. Then he walked next door and started ringing the doorbell until an adult answered and he could ask if Andrew could play.

What kind of solution do you have for that kind of behavior? I don't know the answers, so we got some munchies and sat down to watch Saturday morning cartoons.

Waiting and More Waiting

How was Tom? Did he hurt? Would he come out an invalid? Would he spend the rest of his life in a wheelchair, not able to eat, talk or communicate in any fashion? And the darkest thoughts entered my mind. Would Tom be better if he lived or died? My soul and body hurt. How could I even think that? But they were operating on his brain and the thought was there. I prayed to God and I cursed God. Tom is a kind kid with a wonderful spirit that loves to give and share everything he has with anyone--why him? My thoughts did not really make sense but they swirled with prayers and hope, *"Maybe there is no God, but for today, please be with Tom. Wrap angels around him and give my comfort and peace. I can't be with him, so please, God, take care of my son. Send me to hell, but please be with Tom."*
So many thoughts about life and mortality overwhelmed me. Then the thoughts of how I had failed my son. He had had headaches and we tried to calm him down. When his head hurt and he cried from the pain I would talk him through it, tell him to relax, that he was OK. I would tell him to take breaths, he was dying and I was telling him to breath? We had been to the hospital and doctors' offices no fewer than a dozen times, but did not find a cause for backaches, headaches, and pain. Why didn't I push it? Why didn't I believe in him more, find better doctors, demand tests? There were times I had thought he was faking-- what kind of father am I? Please God and angels, be with Tom.

Basketball

I still feel sick and like an asshole when I think about that day. I wanted to work with Tom and his coach to teach him how to play the game--just the basics. I loved basketball and so did Tom. He would have to be a little close, but he could shoot and make it to a 10 foot rim. We were working on foul shots and he even made me nervous at times that he might beat me at H-O-R-S-E.

Tom was tall for a kid his age--really tall. He was strong and loved basketball. We went down to the school for basketball tryouts. I was sure he was just not trying. He was slow, the last in running lines. He would run to the first, almost come to a complete stop to bend over and touch the line, and then lumber back. I have seen him run with other kids, and with his long legs he could be fast. On this day, he just did not seem to care. I asked him what was going on. He told me he did not know--he was trying. I responded that he was not trying, he probably did not deserve to be on a team, and he needed to put effort into it.

Tom was complaining of headaches and stomach aches, and we took him to the doctor. He underwent CT scans of his abdomen and it showed some gas build up, but no major problems. The doctor suggested, and I agreed, that Tom was experiencing growing pains and was changing. He wanted to sleep more and he was just losing his drive --it happens with kids.

I took Tom jogging with me and he cried. He told me he could not do it and he even fell. I picked him up and held his hand as I pushed him to go. I was sure he was just being a pain to get out of it; all he wanted to do was lie down, watch TV and play video games. We were an active family; we camped, water-skied, played and had fun outside. We were not a TV family. So we just got some headache medication for Tom from the doctor, then headed off for camping in Utah.

After an hour, a nurse came out to let us know that the surgery had begun. That Tom was peaceful and the Dr. Walker was beginning his work. There was a phone in the waiting room and they provided a pager in case we needed to get food or wander anywhere. She told us that she, or one of the doctors, would give us updates as they became available. Then she was gone.

At times we would talk. We would try to reassure each other that Tom was in a good place and in good hands. Children's Primary Hospital is one of the best hospitals in the world and Dr. Walker is the Chief Neurosurgeon. This was the best place for Tom.

Stitches

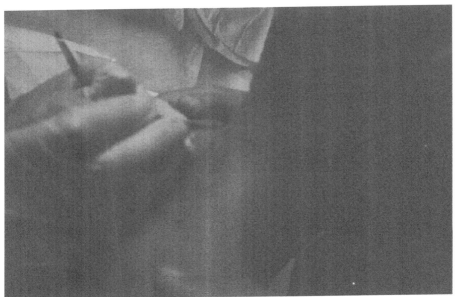

Tom as he is getting the stiches removed from his first brain tumor resection.

I grew up on a small farm, hunting, fishing, raising animals, and all that came with it. I have seen a fair share of blood, including my own. I have witnessed compound fractures and I even witnessed Tom's birth by C-section. Yet all that didn't prepare me for the silly event of watching my son get stitches.

Tom was two when he got his first wound that needed stitching. He has always had energy and a propensity to get into things. At two, he was no different. He simply reached into a kitchen drawer with knives in it and received a deep two and a half-inch cut between his thumb and finger. He screamed and it bled.

I took Tom to his doctor who proclaimed that he needed stitches. The doctor had me hold Tom and keep his hand still while he cleaned and stitched the wound. I was shocked as the doctor inserted the needle through the skin and the room started spinning. I was almost out of control. I was extremely nauseated and had to use all my concentration to stay lucid. I was surprised at the emotions and physical response this little event caused.

The second time Tom received stitches was in the winter of 1992. We lived on a hill in Pleasant Grove, Utah. It was a sunny, cold Saturday, right after a mild snowstorm. We had been waiting for this, so that morning we broke out the sled.

Tom was young and full of energy, but not so much energy that he wanted to keep climbing up the hill after the 45-second slide down. So, soon dad would pull Tom up the hill on the sled and then sled down with him. It was an old fashioned sled with runners, a wood board surface to sit on, and another board perpendicular to the sitting surface was tied to the runners to allow a little steering. After a few trips up the hill, I had the bright idea of tying the rope attached to the sled to our Golden Retriever, Charlie, and letting him pull Tom up the hill. Charlie was large, young and strong and had no problem running up the hill with the sled and kid attached. This method of getting both Tom and the sled up the hill worked well the first few times, and then Charlie spotted a cat under a parked car. Charlie ran directly for the back of the car, as he arrived, the cat ran out to the front and side of the car into the street. The sled, still attached to the dog, followed and crashed into the back of the car. Tom hit the bumper of the car with his face and split his lower lip. The split was severe enough to require stitches, so off to the hospital we went.

The split along the lower line of the lip was likely to scar, so the attending ER doctor called for a plastic surgeon. I held Tom as the surgeon spent his time placing 17 stitches in Tom's lip. The job was done and Tom would survive. We were released with instructions to go to Tom's regular doctor to have the stitches removed in 10 days.

After 10 days I took Tom to the doctor to have the stitches removed. We waited in the reception room, and then we were taken to the patient treatment room to wait for the doctor. When the doctor arrived, he walked past us to the counter, looked at Tom's chart and turned directly toward us. Tom was standing between us looking at the doctor. The doctor looked at Tom and his stitches and said, "Well young man, what happened to you?" Tom looked up at the doctor and replied "My dad thumped me", then turned and looked at me with a big grin. I received a very stern and questioning look from the doctor as I immediately tried to explain about the accident and what really happened. Tom smiled and laughed until the doctor started pulling the stitches. Then I thought about thumping him.

Updates

I don't know how much time went by between updates. The first two were from a nurse. She told us when Tom was under anesthesia, and then when the surgery began, she informed us that everything was going as hoped for. Tom was losing some blood, but that was to be expected. We had signed a waiver for a transfusion if needed. The clock continued to tick.

I thought about Tom. And again the guilt wracked my brain, why had I not made doctors check for a brain tumor sooner? I worried about him dying, and I wondered what he would be like if he lived. Would he be in a vegetative state? Would be restricted to a wheelchair for the rest of his life? Would he ever be able to function on his own? And the worst of all possible thoughts hit me again causing mental anguish accompanied with physical pain, as I wondered which would be worse, living or dying. The hole in my soul continued to grow, the dark pit and darkness seemed to be even darker, if that was even possible. And the fear, oh my god, the paralyzing fear. I had a fear of my own thoughts, a fear of Tom's pain, and a fear of his pain to come. And what about Tom? What really was in his mind? I tried to imagine his thoughts on the trip to the hospital, what he wanted, how he felt, the fear that he must have had and the words he said that haunts me today. My 12 year old son was trying to comfort his father on the way to the hospital. "Dad, it's ok, I'm not afraid to die".

Halfway through the day, Dr. Walker came out for a break and spoke with us. The tumor was indeed large and had caused damage to one side of the cerebellum. There would be long term effects, but we would only know the extent after the surgery and after time. There was still a lot of work to do, but for now Tom was stable. He was a strong kid. Dr. Walker reassured us that kids heal faster than adults do, and Tom had an excellent chance of recovery. The tumor itself did not intrude on the rest of the brain that controls cognitive functions, but the pressure that had built up may have done some damage, possibly significant. We would not know for days. Those days seemed like years.

Full of Life

Tom has always been energetic. He always wanted to help and be a part of everything. When he was three we had just bought our home in Pleasant Grove, Utah, and had decided to add some color and our own touches. Some of the walls in the living room upstairs and adjacent to the glass sliding doors and staircase we had been painting mauve. One day while I was at work, Tom scooted away from his mother. In a very short time, with all his energy and desire to help, Tom painted everything in his reach with mauve paint. He painted the glass doors, the safety rail for the stairs, the fireplace, floor and even some of the appropriate walls. He was so proud and so in trouble. We were both in trouble. Tom's mom wanted to be upset and teach him a lesson. I couldn't stop laughing. What a mess.

When Tom was five, I promised to take him wherever he wanted for food. It was a day for just Tom and me. Tom's mother and I had divorced, and most of the time we spent together included his younger sister, so this was a special occasion. Tom has always been able to eat a great deal and he wanted to go to a place called Mulboone's for their Saturday brunch on the top of a hotel in downtown Salt Lake City.

We dressed up and loaded up. Our plates were stuffed with shrimp, pastries, potatoes, bacon and other various meats. We had plenty of juice and were seated in a booth overlooking the city. Tom finished his plate and wanted more. He asked me to get him some more shrimp and desert. As I left, I gave him a stern warning not to touch anything or get in trouble.

There were four waitresses surrounding Tom and our table when I came back with the food. I had only been gone a minute, what could he have done? Thoughts of the candle being tipped over and the table on fire went through my mind. Thoughts of Tom stabbing someone with his fork. The first words from my mouth were "Tom, what did you do?"

The waitresses were all attractive young women. A young blond waitress immediately came to Tom's defense. She commented on what a great kid he is and the amazing smile. His offense: "He winked at me when I walked by, and I had to tell the others. He is so cute!"

Tom sat there with a huge grin on his face, saying he said he would be good as he began digging into the shrimp. As we finished our meal, the blonde waitress brought our check and I paid with a credit card. We she came back with the receipt, she made a comment about hoping we would return and Tom looked up at her and said "can I have your phone number so we can see you some time?" I was turning a little red as the waitress replied, "I will give it to your dad and you guys can call". She wrote her phone number on my receipt. I regret to say I never called.

A year later when he was six, I had to relocate to Colorado for work so we had all moved to Loveland. We had bought a two level home at the base of Big Thompson Canyon. While on a business trip to Atlanta I received a call from my wife that the basement was flooding. She could not find where the water was coming from, but it was dripping from the ceiling and down the walls. I called a friend to go over and help track down the source and turn the water off to the house. After some investigation, they found that Tom was taking a bath, playing hard and splashing enough water that it went into the heater vents and poured out through three open vents into the basement.

"DAD IT HURTS!"

After surgery Tom was taken into recovery. I was allowed into the recovery room as Tom was waking from the anesthesia. Before I was allowed in, Dr. Walker again addressed our family and let us know that the full tumor was massive and had done significant damage to the right side of his cerebellum, that the hydrocephalus had created a great deal of pressure and possible damage, and he was not sure if Tom would be able to speak or walk.

It seemed like years passed, though it was only minutes or hours; to this day I am still not sure. I had thoughts of what it would be like for Tom, for our family, for me, if he was mentally or physical disabled. What if he would not walk, was forced to live his life in a wheel chair? Could I handle it if he could not think or was mentally retarded? Would he want to live like that? How would I know? What would I do?

I hated myself for even having thoughts like that. He is alive, why was I not just ecstatic? What kind of father was I for even having thought about whether it would be better for my son to live or die? All I should be thinking about is Tom and Amanda, how are my kids, and how can I best support them? But the thoughts still hung in the back of my mind.

The recovery room had lots of activity and two other patients. Several nurses and doctors were treating kids, talking to families, completing paper work, monitoring machines and completing paperwork. Tom's face was swollen from being face down and tilted slightly during his13 hours of surgery. His eyes and mouth were very puffy, almost looking like he had experienced a severe allergic reaction to a bee sting. The next thing that happened was terrible, and wonderful. It haunts me to this day and I am extremely grateful that I was able to experience it. Tom began to awaken from the anesthesia and half screamed, half cried, "DAD, IT HURTS!"

THE IMPORTANCE OF FAMILY

What can you do for the people you love during a time of tragedy? It is amazing how important it is just to show up.

I don't remember asking them to come; truth is I don't remember calling them at all, but within hours my parents, my sister and her husband, and my nephew Jacob were all in the waiting room with me. We shed tears, hugged, and waited together. I am sure we spoke, though I don't know what was said.

My father had served as a Bishop for the Mormon Church. Though I had questioned my own faith for some time I welcomed his offer to give me a Father's Blessing. While I don't remember much of that first day, and I am not good with details, I do remember the soft weight of his hands as he placed them on my head and began to pray.

He prayed to give me strength, peace, and knowledge that God loved me and Tom. He prayed to give me the knowledge and wisdom to make the choices that were coming my way. He prayed to give me the peace and knowledge that I have family who loves Tom and me and that will be there to lift us and hold us, whatever the outcome. In his prayer he told me that he loves Tom and me.

THE DANCE

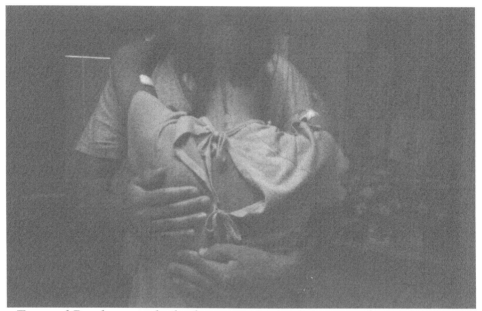

Tom and Randy as we do the dance. He is standing on my feed and holding me as he cries from the pain and frustration

In the few days after his surgery Tom's legs atrophied. His balance was off from the medications, but also from the heavy damage done to his cerebellum, the portion of the brain that controls fine motor skills. Three days after the surgery, he was in severe pain and he could not walk.

The first step was to get him to sit up. A tube sticking out of the top of his head to drain fluid had to be adjusted with each move, to prevent loss of pressure or too much pressure. The 10 inch scar from the crown of his head through the base of his neck showed where skin, muscle and bone were cut away and where pain from each movement originated.

At first he would scream with each movement, but he trusted me-- the doctors and nurses, too, but mostly me--when I told him he needed to do these things to heal. I would put my arm around his shoulders, trusting the others to adjust the levels of the drains and keep the other five IV tubes giving him medicine and life from tangling or pulling. Then he had to stand.

Tom sat on the side of the bed as I crouched down in front of him and he put his arms around my neck. I wrapped my arms under his and around his back, holding him firmly, but as gently as possible. We placed his feet on mine and he began to stand. The effort was enormous. Day one was just that, getting him to stand every two hours.

On the second day we would repeat the same efforts of standing but then we began to teach his legs to move and we began The Dance. We would move slowly around the room with his feet on mine taking small steps, going from one end of the bed to the other. The preparation for each dance seemed to take an hour, but in truth it was about ten minutes. The dance lasted for five minutes at first, then extended with each turn. Those five minutes were brutally exhausting. After each dance he would take more medicine and sleep.

Those first two days seemed to last forever. I was in the room with Tom from the time he got out of surgery. I did not sleep, and sleep would not come for the next five days. My mind was dark and I cried for my son. He would go in and out of sleep with the pain and the medications. He hurt, I was scared, my family and friends were scared, but I had my son, and he could speak.

Chapter 2 - Brain Juice

The brain constantly produces a fluid which fills ventricles in the brain, drains from the head through the spinal canal, and then is absorbed into the body. The growth and trauma of his tumor crushed Tom's natural fluid drainage process, and he would require a shunt. After the initial surgery, an external drain was placed in his head and the fluid drained into a bag hanging on the IV rack next to his bed. The nurses measured the amount of fluid produced and emptied the bag as it filled.

The "brain juice bag" as we had called it, had to be kept at a precise level in relation to his head. If the bag was too high, it would cause excess pressure, not drain well, possibly cause more damage and make his already painful headache worse. If the bag was too low, the fluid would drain too quickly, and cause a great deal of additional pain and dizziness. The precise tool they used to keep the bag level: a yard stick. Each time Tom wanted to roll over, sit up, lay back, or even make a change to his pillow, the nurse would have to check the placement of the bag. Each time we walked, the bag would have to be leveled and walk with us. I was petrified I would make a mistake, fall, trip Tom, or allow some misstep that would rip the drain from his brain.

Post-Surgery Recovery

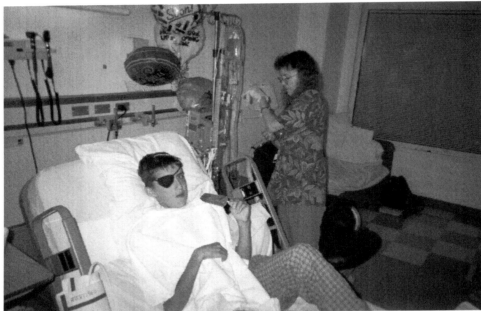

Tom as he recovers at Children's while one of his nurses checks his IV. The eye patch is to force the brain to recognize and use his left eye, the nerves were damaged from the pressure of the tumor.

Children's Hospital in Salt Lake City has a very caring staff of nurses and doctors. It sits on the top of a hill above the University of Utah with views of the Wasatch Mountains and the Salt Lake Valley. They are prepared for critical situations and for parents to stay with their kids. The chair in Tom's room not only reclined, it unfolded almost straight out into a bed. The nurses and aides continually offered me warm blankets, drinks and snacks. They went out of their way to make a very uncomfortable situation comfortable.

The hospital had a library with computer access and a wide range of books and information. At times there would be a volunteer present to help direct, answer questions, or just make conversation, most of the time it was quiet. The halls are all decorated with images from children's stories or toys. They were clean with bright colors, and yet it all felt cold and dim. At times when Tom was sleeping and another family member was there to be with him, I would walk the halls. I would shower in one of the parent's rooms provided and I would try to think, but thoughts, dreams and hopes would not come. All I could do was walk, and focus on what I was doing at the moment and my need to be back where Tom was.

Each day Tom would get up and we would do the dance, teaching his legs to move again. He was young and resilient and his strength came back quickly. It was only a few days until he no longer needed to stand on my feet, but would hold on to me as we took a walk around the bed. In a couple more days, we would be walking into the hall, and then down the hall. It was brutal, still being attached to all the IVs and drains--adjusting, moving, adjusting again--and the pain and energy it took from him was incredible. But despite all this, he made the effort 6 times a day.

On the morning of the 5th day, I was taking Tom for his first walk. My mother-in-law, Cathy, was just outside the room. None of Beth's family had come up for the first days Tom was in the hospital, instead they were welcoming her youngest daughter home from a mission, stayed camping and waited until she had given a talk in church that Sunday in Richfield. They decided to come up after that. I was angry about that. Tom was fighting for his life, Cathy's oldest daughter was in the hospital with her step son, and they decided to wait a few days until after they finished the welcome home and church reception. She knew that I was upset, felt bad, and had come to apologize, maybe explain. I don't know what she would have said, and the timing was wrong when she came to see us. I was walking with Tom and when she asked if she could talk with me I said, "Are you kidding? No!" We never really did talk much after that, though all of Beth's family came to wish him well.

Nurses

Salt Lake City still has a strong influence from the Mormon Church and maintains a heavy family focus and a love of children. Children's Hospital in Salt Lake City was founded by the Mormon Church and was known as Primary Children's Hospital. For many years, the kids in the church would conduct penny drives to help fund the care of other kids--there are many plaques, posters, and works of art around the hospital that honored this. Children's Hospital in Salt Lake City is a teaching hospital attached to the University of Utah. The hospital treats children from all over, kids who are hurting and need a great deal of love as well as medical attention.

Tom was getting better, but he was still in a great deal of pain, and with the pain came opiate based pain medications. One of the side effects of the pain medications is constipation. Getting the bowels moving is also a challenge after surgery so they monitor it closely, and for Tom it was not working. He needed an enema.

Tom was twelve, almost thirteen. He was not shy, but he was going into his teen years and was a bit uneasy. The nurse who came in to administer his enema was a very attractive woman in her early twenties. Tom was hurting, his neck and head in a great deal of pain, and it was a major event just to move so he would not get bed sores. He was trying to be modest, and feeling confused and embarrassed. However, this would be the last time embarrassment would take precedence for him.

The young nurse noticed Tom's hesitation, and I think she was a bit uncomfortable as well. She was kind, and concerned, and wanted Tom to be as comfortable as possible, so she asked him if he would be more comfortable with a male nurse for this procedure. It did not take long for Tom to say yes, and for me to agree, though if you asked him now he would tell you that was a big mistake.

The young nurse made a call and walked out after telling us a male nurse would be there in a few minutes to administer his medication. In a few minutes the door opened and he walked in.

Tom's eyes went wide. He did not say a word. He did not cry, speak, and he barely breathed. This new nurse was young, tall, and thin with short dark hair. He was wearing traditional blue hospital scrubs, and tennis shoes. He was also wearing two small earrings and a bit too much rouge on his cheeks and lipstick. Tom had never experienced a guy dressed like this before. He was shocked and did not know how to react.

He spoke just enough to assure that Tom and the medicine matched up, rolled Tom on his side and administered the enema. He then rolled Tom back, removed his latex gloves, washed and left, saying very little. During this entire time Tom's eyes were wide, his face was turning red, and I don't think he breathed. Once the nurse left and the door was shut he let out a howl. I knew he was hurting, and I should not have laughed, but it just came out. It only lasted for a minute before I was brought back to the pain he was experiencing, but I laughed, and we still laugh at the memory from time to time.

Ronald McDonald House

For the entire time Tom was in the hospital, I stayed in the hospital with him. However, Beth and my parents were there as well. They needed a place to sleep, shower, and re-energize for whatever the next day brought. The Ronald McDonald House welcomed them in. They would take advantage of this hospitality for the next two weeks.

During the time Tom was in the hospital, the Ronald McDonald House charity was conducting a telethon. The producers of the telethon had heard of our story and met Beth at the house. They asked if they could interview us with Tom for the telethon. After talking it through with Tom, we agreed. They came into Tom's room, where we had been staying for over a week by that time, and set up some large cameras and lights. As they talked to Tom, Beth and me, they also took pictures of the banner that kids from home had made for Tom, and the toys, balloons and flowers that covered his room. Tom did well, he smiled, he shared, and he said thank you, and his dad looked pathetic.

The video starts out with an ambulance screaming down the road. Though we were never in an ambulance, it did get the point across. The narration started as the sound of the sirens was dulled and they told about our plan for camping that had turned in to weeks at the hospital with little resources. I have not watched that video in several years, I am not even sure where it is, if it is. The last time I did look at it, the emotions and pain from that day came sweeping over me--it was not fun.

The Ronald McDonald House charged my family $10 a day to stay there. I am still thankful for their help and over the years I have continued to donate to the mission of the house. At a time of complete stress, they succeeded in taking off some of the pressure and some of the pain.

Humbled by Kids

I could see the crash coming but there wasn't anything I could do. It happened quickly, and even though I tried to steer out of it, I went off the road. The bastard hit me, on purpose. He slammed into the back of my car, sent me spinning off the road, and I crashed. It would take a minute, but I knew that a new car with my Donkey Kong character would reappear, and I would head after him for revenge.

Primary Children's Hospital had Nintendo machines on rollers that could be brought into the rooms to play. There were several games, and they did an amazing job of helping to pass the time, and taking Tom's mind off of the pain. Even though he was only twelve, sick, on pain medications, and suffering from what was essentially a major brain injury, he would kick my ass in every game. Except racing. Sometimes.

At times Bug would come in and play, at times a few other people, but he got the most joy out of humiliating his father. I wish I had an excuse, and I did get a little better, but even so, history showed that the beatings would just get worse.

Support

When fumbling my way through these troubled times, I was not aware of the support I would need, or where it would come from. Some of the support was a given--my parents and sister, Michele, were there without question. Steve, my sister's husband, also dropped everything and left work to support Tom and our family. Jacob, my youngest nephew and the cousin closest to Tom's age, insisted on making the cramped, long trip from Sandy, Oregon to Utah. Tom's mother lived in Sandy, Utah, several miles from the hospital, and would come to see Tom almost every day. His step mom, Beth, was there every day with his sister, and so was our dog, Charlie.

Charlie was a 105 lb. golden retriever. He had driven out with us in our 1995 GMC Jimmy and he was relegated to staying in the car for the next two weeks and three days. Beth, my parents and I would take turns visiting the dog, giving him something to eat, and taking him for short walks. He never barked or ran, he waited. Many times I would walk to the car and pet Charlie and he would give me comfort.

I was on vacation from KP Corporation where I was Division President for the Oregon Facility. My boss, Rick, and the Division President for Utah, Dale, came in to visit. I had met Dale several years before when I was working for SoftCopy and he was a vendor, partner with Prolitho. Dale and I were never close friends, at times we were even competitors, and we really did not get to know each other very well. However, Dale, a professional with a pragmatic view on life, came in to visit. I don't remember what either of them said. I imagine it was words of comfort, not to worry about work and to call if I needed anything. What I do remember is Dale, a strong, opinionated business manager, with tears in his eyes, giving me a hug and tells me he would pray for Tom and my family.

My team back in Salem, Oregon would call each day and ask for updates and send their thoughts and prayers. They put a care package together for Tom and talked to him at times on the phone. My operations manager, Tony, sent along a video for Tom, Happy Gilmore. Happy Gilmore is an irreverent Adam Sandler movie that I am not sure I would give to a 12 year old boy. However Tony had great insight, Tom loved it and it is still one of his favorite movies today. Thanks Tony.

The First Trip Out

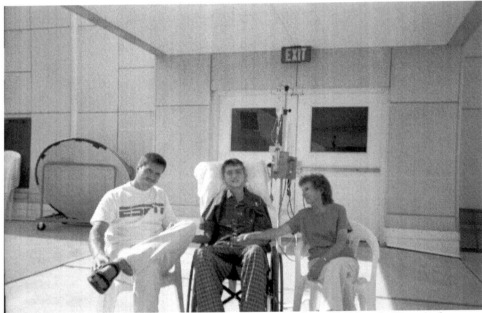

Tom's first day outside after surgery in Salt Lake City Children's Hospital.

Each day Tom got stronger, and it became evident that he was going to make it through this. He still could not walk far on his own, and it had been more than a week since he had been outside. It was August in Utah. His first venture outside was in a special wheelchair designed to support people with neck injuries. It was still difficult just to get him from the bed to the chair.

Tom, like me, was a sun nut. He loved the water, could water-ski and kneeboard, loved camping and getting dirty. When he was seven, he was riding in the bow of our small boat as it was time to head home. We were going very slowly and he was complaining that he wanted to swim some more, he did not want to go home, the sun was still out. I told him to knock off the whining and I turned to look at something in the back of the boat. When I turned back around all I could see was one of Tom's hands holding onto the rail on the front of the boat, he had jumped over, but decided to hold on because the boat was moving. I turned off the engine and pulled him in; he is too hard-headed to have fear.

Children's Hospital had a small roof top area for patients, medical staff, and family to get some outside air. This was our first venture into the sun. We had been able to replace the hospital gown with long plaid pajama bottoms and a casual, blue button up silk shirt. Once we got Tom into the chair, the brain juice bag had to be connected to the stand connected to the chair. Then the other IV bags had to be moved and the electronic monitoring devices had to be disconnected. This process took about ten minutes and left Tom exhausted before we got out of his room.

The trip down the hall and into the elevator had to be navigated with care. I had to repress my desire to do wheelies with the chair--that would come later. Each bump had to be taken slowly, each movement came with tense anticipation of shock and pain. The movement of the elevator was not received with joy.

My mom and Beth accompanied us outside on that first trip. The sun was warm and bright and it felt good to me. Tom wanted to be outside, wanted the fresh air and the warmth, wanted so badly to be out of the hospital--and then reality set in. It was the sun. The sun that we so loved. The time of year where we would wait for it to come up so we could rush out and play in the water. The sun quickly became Tom's enemy. From the pressure, surgery and trauma to the brain, Tom had become extremely sensitive to light. With all of the tubes and sensitivity he could not wear sunglasses, though at this point they would do little good. The sun that was drawing us out, giving energy, creating desire, was also hurting my son and drove us back into the safety of the hospital.

As a father the emotions were exceptional, the joy overwhelming. The fear and darkness persisted, but if felt like the first time I had been able to breathe in days. Almost as if I had been trapped under water, suffocating, panicked that I was going to drown, and then catching my first breath. The tears of joy began to pour, and there was not a damn thing I could do about it, and at that moment I did not care.

Better Each Day

A new nurse walked in that we had not met and it started all over again. "Do you know the difference between Deer Nuts and Corn Nuts? Corn Nuts are usually 75 cents and Deer Nuts are just under a buck." Tom had a set of jokes that he tried out on everyone he met. By now, his room was full of handmade posters, cards, books, flowers, cookies and candy, and an abundance of pretty much everything that can be sent to a kid's hospital room. Tom was a big fan of John Stockton and the Utah Jazz. His mom had called the Jazz and asked if players ever visited sick kids and if one would come and visit Tom. She was told they were getting ready for the season, focused, and would not be able to send anyone over, but they did send posters, pictures and a small purple basketball that was proudly displayed in his room.
Tom was getting stronger each day; the recovery was really quite amazing. He still ran out of energy too quickly and had a great deal of pain, but he was laughing, telling jokes, walking farther, and healing. Everyone laughed, or at least rolled their eyes at his jokes. Dr. Walker had come to check on Tom and told us that the pathology reports had come back, and that Tom's tumor was an astrocytoma. This was good news. Originally, with the size and growth patterns, he thought it was a much worse type of tumor, and our goal was to keep Tom alive for five years as new treatments and methods were being found.

Astrocytoma tumors grow very slowly, or not at all, for long periods of time. Childhood brain tumors are uncommon but this type of tumor is not usually malignant and does not spread. His tumor was large and had a core. It had been removed, and was not expected to come back. Things were rough, but they were going to be OK. If you are going to have a brain tumor as a kid, this was a fairly easy one to treat. Soon we would be going home.

Before we could go home, though, the 28 staples that held the skin together on the back of Tom's head needed to be removed. The scars started at the crown of his head and traveled to the base of his neck. There was a much smaller scar on the top of his head where the shunt was placed, and small scars along his neck and abdomen where the tube traveled down to let the fluid drain into his abdomen. A young doctor, a resident in neurosurgery, came in to remove the stitches.

The doctor talked to Tom and examined his head. Tom sat the side of his bed and the doctor was behind him. Tom's head needed support so I stood in front of him and held his head, his face in my chest. Tom did great and the doctor removed the staples with little bleeding, but for me it started again. Standing there, holding my son, the world seemed to be spinning wrong. The room seemed to get hot and I began sweating. The process took just a few minutes but it took all I had to stand there with Tom, but I could not let him go. I could not let him see that this was tough for me, he had to be tough, and he is my son, no one else should be there. This would be one of the most difficult times in my life I have had, trying to control my body and keep from falling. After several minutes, the staples and stitches were gone, Tom lay down, and I fell into a chair to breathe and regain my composure.

Chapter 3 - Her Name is Bug

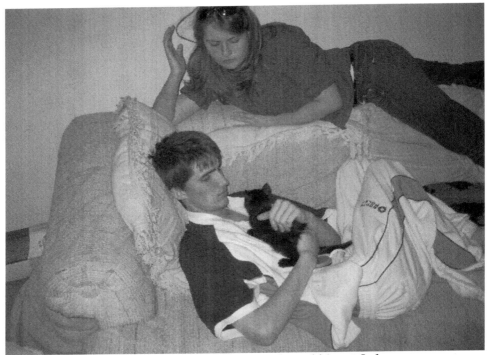

Tom recovering at home with his sister Amanda and his cat Jade

Her name is Amanda, but I call her Bug. Every morning she would come in with her mom into Tom's room and then head off to the children's play room. I had walked with her to the play room a couple times, but never really spent much time there. I am not sure what I was thinking. Probably that I had to be with Tom, and that she would understand, or at least, needed to learn to understand. It would be years before I learned how she felt, how the time we missed was much more than I could comprehend. Even though there were events, and signs, that this was affecting her deeply.

I have called her Bug, or Buggy, as long as I can remember. Today she is a beautiful woman studying to become a nurse, something she has focused on since elementary school. Back then she was only eight years old. Every morning she would come to the hospital with her mom, see Tom and then head to the play room. On this particular morning, she arrived right at 7:30 am, right at shift change. During shift change everyone was asked to leave Tom's room, including me, for 30 minutes. The nurses would get together to talk about the patients, and family, and what care they needed. Bedding would be changed and then we could return.

Bug came to see her brother but she had to wait for 30 minutes, and she immediately broke down crying. She was scared, hysterical, screaming she wanted to see her brother, why couldn't she see Tom? I tried to explain that the nurses were changing and we could go in shortly, but she would not be calmed. I was unprepared for this. I did not know what to do, so I just held her and waited.

At the end of the shift change, I took Bug in to see Tom. She immediately calmed down, and within minutes was ready to go out on an adventure. She had a small basket that she took around the hospital. I think she stopped at every nurse's station, and person she could find, to collect treasure, and brought Tom back a "Treasure Chest" to help him feel better.

Hey Dad, So this is what I remember.
Tom was sick, throwing up, crying, and falling over. You grabbed Beth and drove him to a hospital. I was walking around, exploring, when you came back to the campsite. You were pale, Beth told me to grab my bag and get in the car. When I asked what was happening, you just told me that Tom was really sick and needed to see the doctor. The car ride felt like it took forever. When we got to the hospital, there were a lot of people. I remember going in to the main lobby and seeing a big sculpture of something. I don't remember what, only that it seemed to fill the room. I remember Beth taking me to get something to eat while Tom was in getting an MRI with you. The cafeteria was very plain. Nothing too special, but I can remember the smell of the food cooking, and the look of all the staff. We met you in a waiting room of sorts, you said Tom was really sick and had to go in for surgery. The look on your face was possibly the scariest thing I'd ever seen. Before that day, I had never seen you cry. I remember when Mom came up and how despite your differences, Tom was all that mattered. I remember when Grandma and Grandpa came up. I also remember going with Beth to the Ronald McDonald house and seeing a quilt that was made for the families of the patients. I remember the one male nurse who helped Tom after his surgeries. He was nice, and he would walk me to the kids room every once in a while. I remember when Tom went in for surgery. Dr. Walker was really nice. Everyone was quiet. They all put on happy faces for me, but I remember seeing the fear in everyone, and trying not to be afraid myself. To be honest, I remember trying to be brave, because if Tom could do it, I could too. I wasn't about to let my older brother show me up! ;)

When the surgery was over, I remember seeing the relief spread over everyone's faces. I know the prospect of Tom never being able to walk or talk again was scary, but he made it through the surgery and that was what's important. The next few days were kind of blurry, I was usually in the kids room, whether that was because I was in the way, or just to keep me busy, I don't know. I remember a boy though, he had cancer too. His head was shaven, he was a year younger than me, and he had been there for quite some time. He let me play Donkey Kong with him. I was the little monkey. He told me how everyone was really nice, and that they made him feel much better. He also helped me make pictures for Tom. I think it was that little boy who taught me hope.

I remember when Tom had to start walking around again. It was scary seeing him cry and shout. It was also scary seeing the large scar in the back of his head. I was mad at the doctor because I thought it was his fault Tom was hurting. I remember Tom playing lots of video games, and you, Mom, and Beth all in the room. I remember when the video was made and you were interviewed. I remember making Tom a picture of a fish using paper pieces. I also remember wishing I could go into the big kid's room because there were cool games in there. I also remember Tom going in for another MRI. I gave him my favorite blanket. It was pink with a ton of Sylvester the Cat pictures on it. I had had it since I could remember. The nurse told me I would probably not get it back, but I wanted Tom to have something from home, so I said that was okay. Today, I like to think that it still helps make the hospital a little less scary for a child.

I remember Tom slowly getting better. He would tell jokes, flirt with the nurses, and bully me as usual. I also remember being forced to go back to school. Tom was still in the hospital, but I had to go to 4th grade. I was not happy about leaving. My teachers were nice, though. They were lenient with homework and helped me when I would get worried. I remember lots of car rides back and forth. I also remember the layout of Tom's room. He was against the wall, a TV with game console in front of him, a sink to the left of his bed (if facing him), the recliner chair you usually sat in, and the couch in the corner under the window. You also slept in a parent's room during the surgery (I think it was because Beth made you). Everyone took turns babysitting me, but I pretty much had the run of the hospital, and the staff didn't seem to mind. They knew who I was and where I went if I got lost (which happened a couple times). The last thing I remember was Tom being released from the hospital. It was a good day, one that had us all smiling. That was probably the scariest experience, being told I might lose my brother. But to be honest, I don't remember crying. I know no one really thinks about what I remember, or what I saw, but I watched you and everyone else very closely. I knew exactly what was happening, but it was my job to be a little girl, and I think that was what I needed to do. I was a distraction, and I was okay with that. When the family was busy with me, it didn't give them time to worry about Tom. It may sound selfish, but I didn't like seeing my family cry.

These events were not only life changing and painful for a son and his dad, they had a very profound effect on a daughter and sister. The scars are deep, and after more than a dozen years, they still bleed tears.

Chapter 4 – Family

It was late in the afternoon. I was 16, and I had never seen my mom that mad. I really had not done anything wrong--at least, nothing she actually knew of. I was just late, she did not know where I was, and she was worried. She stood there yelling at me and hitting me as hard as she could over and over… with a pink fuzzy slipper. Though I tried not to, all I could do was laugh, and pretty soon she was laughing too.

My niece gave her the name "Chocolate Grandma", because she almost always has chocolate close at hand. Her favorite is See's candies, and if she has a pound, you can be sure of two things: one, that if you turn them over, the bottom of each piece will be broken open to visually inspect what kind of filling is inside, and two, that those chocolates will be gone in less than 24 hours. A small woman — all of 5'2" when she stretches out on her toes, and normally weighing close to 105 pounds — with a great big heart, this is Charlotte, my mom, Tom's grandmother.

Though very opinionated, she almost always has a smile. She has a strong faith in God, is very active in her church, teaches Sunday school, and is loved by almost everyone. She has a special place in her heart for all kinds of animals. Once, one of her cats caught a small squirrel, and she rushed out to take the small animal away from the cat, and then nursed that squirrel back to health until it was well enough to be released. She feeds the birds daily, and cries when one of them dies from hitting one of the large picture windows in the front of their home.

Ray, my father, and Tom's Grandpa, is 5'11" with a large bark and a deep, caring heart. A retired firefighter, he worked part time as a truck driver until we moved to a rural area several miles from the closest town, where he built a house, barn, and a small farm. Having served as a Bishop in the Mormon Church, he has also spent a great deal of time volunteering and helping members of the community. He cares much less about what religion you are, or even if you believe in God, than about helping when he sees a need. He still works on other people's cars when they need help, build things, and makes sure he is with those in time of need. There is no question, he just goes. He is the patriarch of his family and his dedication to their wellbeing is enormous.

Three years older than me, my sister Michele is always working on a social cause. A mother of five, she has testified in Salem, Oregon on the need for stronger laws controlling the distances that strip clubs, bars, and other adult entertainment centers can be located next to schools. She has fought for her belief in the right to life, and champions care for the mentally ill. Michele always has a cause and is an extremely driven woman. She is supported by her husband Steve.

It was about 2:00 in the afternoon on August 16, 2000 when I called my dad at his home. We had arrived at Children's Hospital in Salt Lake City about 30 minutes before, and Tom had already had a hole drilled in his skull to relieve the pressure. No one remembers the exact words that we said, but by the time they hung up the phone, my parents were already making preparations to drive over 700 miles to be with us.

Mom was terrified. All she could think of was "let's go" and all she could feel was fear and worry for all of us. A brain tumor and emergency surgery? Is Tom dying? Would he be alive when they got there? We have to leave now.

Dad can get upset if the check book is out of balance by $5, or if one of the grandkids makes a snide remark. At times he will raise his voice or become irritated by seemingly small things, but in times of real emergency he is calm, and takes charge of his surroundings and the wellbeing of those around. After I hung up and he talked to my mom, he called Michele, told them they were headed to Utah, and she immediately said she was leaving work. They were all on the way toward us.

Dad doesn't remember much about the actual trip. It started with a prayer, asking for strength and comfort for all of our family and protection for Tom. They left, and drove through the night. The exit to Multnomah Falls off I-84 is an odd one. Taking off on the left, it looks like the exit lane goes straight as the freeway turns slightly to the right. Doing over 70 MPH, dad accidently took the exit and drove through the parking lot without hesitation or slowing--he was focused.

They arrived at the hospital early the next morning after a twelve hour drive. Tom was already in surgery, and mom rushed in and threw her arms around me, crying and asking me if I was OK. Dad hugged me and Beth, and asked if we were OK, and how Tom was. Michele, Steve and Jacob did the same. Dad gathered us together and offered a prayer, and then we all watched the second hand on the clock move as we waited.

Slurpee Please

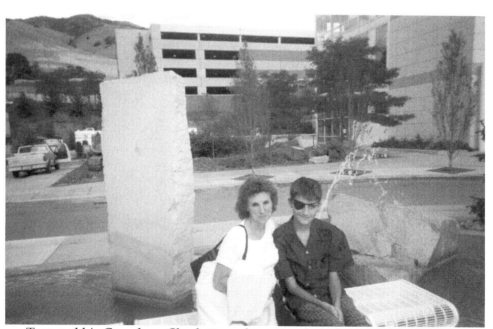

Tom and his Grandma, Charlotte, as he get ready to leave Children's in Utah and head home to Oregon.

Mom and 7-Eleven should almost have their own chapter. Every morning on the way to the hospital from the Ronald McDonald House, mom and Beth would take a detour to get Tom a Slurpee. There would be a request for another one twice more during the day, every day. His favorite was a mixture of Coke and cherry flavors, but at times he would get other flavors as they were available. The Slurpee became a comfort food for Tom, a sign of love and as important as many of the medications.

Mom has seven grandkids, but Tom has always had a very special place in her heart. He was always just a bit mischievous, and ornery, but with a big smile that melted her heart. She would get him anything, and she made damn sure he had a Slurpee when he needed it. Other than to sleep, she hardly left his side, or mine. She would not have left even then, but only one person was allowed to spend each night with Tom, and each night, that was me. She understood, but I don't think she was happy about it.

Mom was not feeling well on the trip to Salt Lake City. She had been concerned for a while, and had been thinking that she really should see a doctor, but for now that would wait. There were more urgent matters to attend to and her family needed her.

Tom continued to walk further each day, and gain strength. The corny jokes got cornier and the thrashing of his dad in video games became more frequent. With all he had been through, he was still concerned about others. When the video console was brought into his room, he would ask if one of the other kids needed it. He was concerned about me and my job, "Dad, you can go home and work if you need to, I understand." As long as he had his Slurpees he was going to survive.

Towards the end of his stay at the hospital a social worker asked Tom to talk with another kid in the hospital, a young girl who had been diagnosed with a brain tumor and was extremely frightened. Tom agreed and the social worker wheeled Tom into her room. He spent some time with her telling her how great the doctors are and assuring her that she would be OK. He told her about his adventure and that he had almost died, but they took care of him, she was in the right place. When it was time to go back to his room, he asked for more pain medication as his smile faded. That was tough.

Home

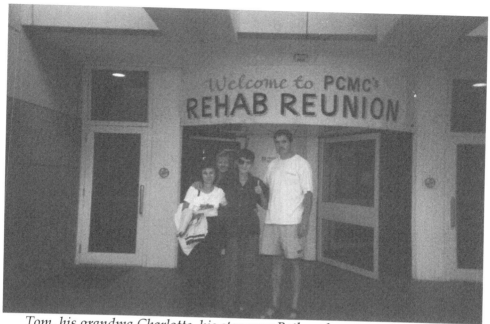

Tom, his grandma Charlotte, his stepmom Beth and me as we leave Children's hospital and head for home.

Tom was improving, and after two weeks, it was getting close to time to go home. Tom, Beth, Bug and I had arrived at the hospital with our dog Charlie in a red GMC Jimmy. Mom, dad, Michele, Steve and Jacob had made the trip in a Ford Crown Victoria. Bug would be staying with her mom in Utah.

We had plenty of room in our vehicles for the drive home, but the trip through the mountains would be difficult for Tom. We were concerned about Tom's comfort on a long car trip, with the changes in pressure, and, of course, the miles between 7-Elevens for Slurpees. We decided that Tom should fly back to Oregon. Who would make the plane trip with Tom? There was little question about that—it would be Grandma. Dad, Michele, Steve and Jacob took my SUV with the dog a few days early so they could meet the plane, and take Tom home. Beth and I waited with mom for Tom to be released.

Tom was released from the hospital 16 days after we had arrived. He was fitted with a neck brace, and we spent the last night at the Marriot Hotel close to the hospital. We took plenty of time to get up the next morning and prepare for the trip home. We got into the car and headed to the Salt Lake City airport, making a stop at 7-Eleven. Once at the hospital, I found a wheel chair with a neck support and we headed for the gate. It was a tense day for me. There was relief for my son being out of the hospital and on his way home, and there was tension because I did not think the airline staff was giving Tom and mom the attention they needed. There was the anxiety of being separated from my son after all that had transpired over the past few weeks. But Tom and mom got on the plane, and Beth and I watched it take off, before heading back to the car and speeding back to Oregon.

The doctors had given Tom some muscle relaxers and pain medication that made him sleepy. His body was also worn out from the surgery, which was essentially brain trauma, and the harsh recovery. Fortunately, the weather was good and the flight back to Oregon in early September was an uneventful one.

Thinking back on that plane trip, Mom recalls, "We talked a little and Tom told me he hurt. He laid his head on my lap and slept most of the way. This whole time I felt so helpless, there was so little I could do. He is so precious and does not deserve this. I wish I could take this away."

I don't remember much about my own car trip back across Utah, Idaho, and Oregon to get home. I do remember being tired, having just discovered that I could live for more than 5 days without sleep. Somewhere along the way, Beth and I talked about the changes we were going to have to make to care for Tom, what he would need, and how we would provide it. There was still fear, too, about what Dr. Walker had initially said. In his first trip out of the operating room, he told us that the shape and pattern of Tom's tumor made him think it was cancerous, and a very aggressive form. Although the pathology report returned later with a much more promising story, those first words still haunted me. Somehow, even then, despite Tom's improved prognosis, I knew we were in for a rough ride. I was wondering how I would find the best care for my son.

Chapter 5 – Charlie

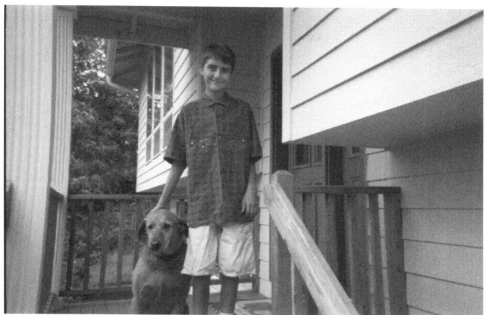

Tom's return home to Salem, Oregon with his dog Charlie.

It was late spring, 1991. Tom was three, and he and I had gone out to Kroger's to do some shopping. I don't remember what we needed at the store, but the day is difficult to forget. Impulse buying is a specialty of grocers, and on this particular day, it seemed to follow us out the door.

Just outside the Kroger's in Orem, Utah, sat a young boy, no older than ten, and his mother. Beside them was a large, brown cardboard box that contained a large, reddish brown puppy with paws that were definitely too big for him and floppy ears. Tom, being three, and me, just being me, had to stop and pet the puppy. The boy was heartbroken. I talked to the mom, and she told me that they were moving across country and could not take the puppy with them--they had to give it away.

I don't know what I was thinking; we already had a dog, a medium sized lab. This guy was already big, and he was only 11 weeks old. Tom was three, Bug was just an infant, and we had absolutely no need for another dog. So, naturally, we took the puppy and gave the kid $25 for spending money on their trip. What else could we do?

Charlie, as we decided to name him, was a short haired golden retriever with a LOT of energy.

He came home with us to our four bedroom house in Pleasant Grove, Utah. The house had a good sized back yard surrounded by a five foot cyclone fence. The backyard featured a large, old apricot tree with a raised bed around it, and a giant boulder over in the corner where the fence curved around. Down the hill, just three blocks from the house, was an irrigation canal with a gravel road that ran along each side. On the far side of the canal was an apricot orchard. The canal ran for miles, and I never did learn where it started or where it ended. It would fill and drain at different times of the year, presumably when the farmers had a need for irrigation.

Charlie was an extremely hyperactive young dog who needed a great deal of attention. He loved everyone, and his favorite way to express his love was by jumping up and licking you on the face. It seemed he would only sit still when he was sleeping. Tom would run after him, sometimes pulling on his tail, ears or feet. Charlie would nudge Tom, paw at him, and put his mouth on his arms and legs, never biting hard, and Tom would laugh.

Charlie grew quickly and I bought him a large wooden dog house, with the intention of keeping him outside. When he did come in, he seemed to bring large bags of dirt and mud with him, to spread around the house. Pam was not happy with it, but she tolerated it. Kind of. Bug was too small to notice much, and Charlie was too hyper to spend much time checking out the infant.

Our water meter at the house was just inside the fence, and as Charlie grew, the meter reader became nervous of him. Charlie would frequently bark at him when he came to put his probe over the fence to read the water usage. The trash collector was quite different.

Once a week I would set the trash out on the corner by the fence, and the collector would come and pick it up. I never heard complaints about Charlie barking at the trash man, and though it seemed odd, I did not give it much thought. Late one morning I was home, and Charlie was inside with me when the trash man came. As the truck was coming up the street, Charlie ran to the back door and wanted out. He whined, paced back and forth, and was very anxious. I let him out and he ran around the house to the corner to meet the trash man. It occurred to me what he was doing, so I put on shoes and took off after him. As I got to the corner I saw Charlie, now about 80 lbs., standing on his hind feet with his front paws on the top of the fence. I realized that he could jump the fence and hoped that he would not. The garbage truck stopped and Charlie barked. The trash man came around the truck, took off his gloves and rubbed Charlie's head. I said hello, introduced myself, and apologized if the dog was giving him concerns. He laughed as he reached in his pocket for a treat for Charlie, and said "No, I love this dog".

I began running that summer, to help build endurance for water-skiing. I would take Charlie and we would run down the hill, past a large German Shepherd that barked, growled, and strained at his chain to chase after us, over to the canal, and then along the canal for a mile or two. Then we'd turn around and run back the canal, up the hill, past the shepherd and back to the house. We would do this three or four times a week, almost every week.

I think Charlie was close to a year old when my neighbor Les decided to run with me. I had decided not to take Charlie this time, and left him in the back yard. We were running down the hill, less than a block away when Charlie ran, jumped, hit the top of the boulder in the corner of the yard, and used it to spring over the fence with little effort. He was determined to run with us. This became a regular occurrence. I would go running and Charlie would jump the fence to run with me. To my knowledge he never jumped the fence any other time.

One evening, Pam and the kids were gone when I arrived home; Charlie was in the back yard. A police car drove up to my driveway and stopped. The officer got out and rang my doorbell. The officer introduced himself and asked if the dog was friendly. I said yes and Charlie walked up to him to say hi. The officer played with Charlie while asking me what kind of dog he was, how long we had had him, and if we had received any complaints about him. I gave him the information, told him we had never had a complaint, and asked why he was inquiring about complaints. The officer told me that the water meter reader wanted his probe back. It seems that Charlie took the probe as the reader was reaching over the fence and then became protective and would not let him retrieve it. That had never happened before and never happened again.

Charlie was now almost two and we were running along the canal. We frequently saw ducks swimming in the canal, and they would fly off as we got close, or dive under the water. On this particular day, Charlie saw the ducks before I did, and he took off. He jumped from the side of the canal into the water, and three of the ducks flew off, the fourth dove in. Bad call. The duck could only swim one direction, and Charlie was swimming after it. The duck looked up, saw the dog and dove in again, but eventually he could not keep that up, and Charlie caught his duck.

I called Charlie, nervous that he had killed a duck, wondering what to do. Charlie came right to me, very proud, and dropped the duck at my feet. The duck was not dead, but it did not move much either. I had Charlie sit, and held him as we watched the duck regain its senses, and fly off. We had passed many ducks swimming in the canal before and, after that day, we passed many more without incident. Obviously that particular duck has dissed him.

On another day along the canal, we saw our neighbor's German Shepherd just as we were finishing our run and heading back up the hill. As usual, he was barking and straining at his leash to get to us. Charlie was about fifty yards ahead of me, parallel to the German Shepherd, when he stopped and looked back at me. He hesitated for a moment, looked back at the shepherd, and then took off running at him as fast as he could. Charlie collided with the other dog at full speed, and the two dogs tumbled over each other. There was a brief exchange of fighting before Charlie rejoined me for the run, as if nothing had happened. We ran past this dog hundreds of times before and since, and he never did that again. As he got older, Charlie would play with the kids, fetch tennis balls, and ignore sticks. He would follow Tom around, and both Tom and Bug would crawl all over him. He mellowed out, and would lie next to me as I petted him. However, as soon as I stopped the movement of my hand, he would nudge me with his nose.

In 1993, Pam and I split up, and I moved to Arizona for work. I lived in a three bedroom house with my friend Michael, and another roommate, Hans. I was only there for a short time, when Pam called to tell me she was taking Charlie to the pound. Michael and I immediately drove to Pleasant Grove to pick up Charlie, and bring him to Arizona.

Michael and Hans were single, I was getting divorced, and Charlie was a chick magnet. Everyone loved Charlie, and he loved everyone. However, he hated Michael smoking. Every time Michael lit a cigarette Charlie would walk away.

I did not stay in Arizona very long before making another move — this time, to Loveland, Colorado. I bought a large house in Loveland, close to a long, paved running trail at the mouth of the Big Thompson Canyon. The long and winding road though the steep cliffs of the Big Thompson Canyon runs along the Big Thompson River and leads to Estes Park, and the Rocky Mountain National Park. From the outside, the house looked average in size, but inside was a 1600 square foot main floor with a full finished basement of the same size. The master bedroom was on the main floor with its own large bathroom and walk-in closets. There were also three bedrooms upstairs and a fifth down stairs. Most of the basement was a large play room.

Pam and I decided to get back together, so she and the kids moved into the house in Loveland with me. It was rocky, but good to have my family back. It also did not last long. Pam went back to Utah, and I took some time off from work to stay at home with Tom, Bug, and Charlie.

There is not much good about getting divorced, but I do have very fond memories of having time to stay at home with the kids. Nothing amazing happened--no great, terrible or funny events, just a peaceful time playing with the kids and the dog. We would sit on the porch in the evening and watch the lightning as the summer thunder storms would build in the mountains. We biked, swam, played and went boating. Too soon, the kids returned to Utah to stay with Pam. But even that arrangement did not last long, and Tom returned to Colorado to live with Charlie and me.

Tom had a great deal of energy and was tough for his mom to handle. He looks a lot like me, enough to evoke frequent comments. He had also adopted quite a few of my quirks and habits, even at a young age. All this led Pam to complain constantly about his behavior, and agree that Tom was better off living with his dad and his dog.

While I was in Colorado, I met and married Beth. Not long after, I took a new job in Fife, Washington, and Tom, Beth, Charlie, and I were again on the move. We found a modest three bedroom home in North Tacoma, just five miles from my office. Charlie and I would run around the neighborhood for exercise, Tom attended elementary school five blocks from the house, there were local kids Tom's age to play with, and life was good.

Charlie was great at staying with me while we ran, and I often ran with him off leash. Four blocks down from our house was a family that owned a Siamese cat. The cat would often arch its back and hiss as we ran by. I would take care that Charlie did not go after it. Charlie just ignored the cat. One morning, on the way past the house, the owners of the cat were out, and we chatted. It was a man and a woman, in their thirties, fit and seemingly happy. I told them about running by and introduced them to Charlie. The laughed a bit when I expressed concern that Charlie might chase the cat. They commented that it was one tough cat, still had all its claws, and has been known to fight and beat dogs over territory. They were not worried.

It had been several months since I had met the owners of the cat, and we had run past it many more times. Then one day we were running, the cat was hissing, and Charlie paused. I had seen this once before, and now, just as then, there was nothing I could do about it. Charlie was off like a bat out of hell. The cat stood its ground, and Charlie scooped it up while still at full speed and threw it in the air, and against the house. The cat came down and took off around the house, eventually running up a tree. Charlie did not give chase, but came back to finish our run as if nothing had happened.

We were still living in Tacoma when Beth went to Utah to visit her family. I was running along the edge of the neighborhood, and Charlie was on a leash since it was a fairly busy road. I saw the small, red Toyota MR2 coming through the side street. It was slowing down for the stop sign as we kept pace through the intersection. The driver was looking the opposite direction and saw a car coming; she was turning with traffic and could beat it if she hurried, so she stepped on the accelerator. Charlie stopped and pulled back on his leash. The car hit me with its right front panel, about fifteen inches into the hood. I was thrown on top of the car, collapsing the roof, and breaking the front windshield and passenger window. I came down on top of Charlie. When all was done, I had dislocated my right hip, had some significant bruising, and Charlie had two broken ribs. We were done running for a while.

Charlie developed a growth on the right side of his nose, what appeared to be a wart. We tried some over the counter wart medicine but the sore kept growing and getting larger, until it was the size of a quarter. I had had Charlie for about eight years and he had become a friend and companion to my family and I, so we took him to the vet to get him checked out. It took just a short time for the veterinarian to inform us that our dog had cancer. She referred us to another veterinarian who specialized in cancer in animals.

The specialist informed us that Charlie needed surgery to remove the tumor. He would remove the part of the tumor that we saw and continue removing the affected flesh and bone until all the cancer was gone. It would be rough on the dog, he could not guarantee the outcome, and it would cost just over $1000. The good news was it did not appear to be overly invasive yet, and Charlie was a young and fit dog. We felt that we had no choice and we opted for the surgery.

Charlie came out of the surgery with a cone on his head to protect the wound. The cancer had invaded into his nasal area and some cartilage and a fair amount of the flesh on his left side were removed. It was tough on Charlie but he did heal, though he looked happy from this right and like he was permanently growling on his left. The whole event was tough and would take him months to recover from, but recover he did; we had our dog.

After living in Tacoma for four years it was time to move again. I was offered a position of Division President for K/P Corporation in Salem, Oregon. I was to take over the original K/P facility and team, a small printing company along the Willamette River. Beth was excited to look for a new home. She loved looking at houses, going to the Parade of Homes, and experiencing the draw of new and different things.

We thought hard about what we wanted: a house with a basement, close to work, a big master bathroom, a garage big enough for the boat, privacy, and a few other specifics that I don't recall. Beth had gotten online and had a large list of homes to go see. She had spoken with a realtor and was prepared for three solid days of house shopping.

Salem, the capitol of Oregon, is a small town of about 150,000 in the Willamette Valley, built along the Willamette River. Most of the town and businesses are on the east side of the river, including K/P, which was a ½ mile from the bridge. The west side of the river is mostly homes. We were looking for a home on the west side one day, when we got lost. I needed to turn around, and there was a gravel driveway with a for sale sign on the side, that I decided to use. When we pulled up the driveway, we saw a new home and a worker hosing off the cement parking pad. We spoke to the worker for a few minutes and learned that his brother was the contractor. This was a 2/3 acre lot built into the side of a hill. On the other side of the lot was a cherry orchard. The driveway was part easement and it was ¼ mile long.

The builder let us walk through the house. He told us that they were just getting ready to list it, as he showed us around. It had everything we had put on our list, was within our price range, and was ready to move into. The builder gave us his brother's contact information and we drove over to meet him. Beth was devastated, excited, and conflicted. We could not buy the first house we saw! She had a long list of places to see. But we both knew this was going to be our home, and we ended up only looking at one more place.

We found a realtor in Tacoma and began the process of selling our old house. The realtor had been in the house several times and had gotten along great with Charlie. Then the call came. We were out one Saturday afternoon and had left Charlie inside. It was dusk and the realtor had stopped by to put some things in the house for a showing the next day. As he tried to open the door, Charlie stood his ground, protective and growling, not letting anyone in. We made sure to take Charlie with us the next day for the open house, where we did in fact find a buyer.

Tom, Beth, Charlie and I all moved to Salem, Oregon, into the house adjacent to the cherry orchard. This was the home we brought Tom back to, after that excruciating trip to Utah. It was now September, 2000 and Tom was home to heal. Charlie had become a close friend to both Tom and me and provided an unforeseen emotional support to us both.

Chapter 6 – Void of Light

Tom was afraid to get on the plane. He was mostly afraid of the takeoff and landing. He had flown before and even at twelve he knew about the pressure changes and turbulence. He head hurt, his neck hurt, and he was afraid the flight would hurt. He was done hurting, but what else could he do? Driving would take much longer, be bumpier, and he would still feel the pressure of the mountains. And he had to go home with dad and Beth, staying with mom was not even a thought. Tom had complete faith in his dad; dad would make the right decisions, and make everything OK. The flight was not nearly as bad as he thought it might be. The neck brace dad bought helped, and he really did not feel the pressure much. He had slept on grandma's lap, though he did not remember falling asleep, nor waking up, just that it was time to land. Thank god the landing was smooth and the trip seemed mostly like any of the others he had been on. Grandpa was there waiting to pick them up.

What an excruciating adventure. We were finally back at home at our house in Salem, Oregon. What started out as a gathering with Beth's family, and my birthday, had become a nightmare, but we made it. Tom was still hurting, but happy to be home. It was a warm September day when we arrived and Tom was smiling. At the age of twelve he was already close to six feet tall, skinny, and sporting a magnetic grin. He had his dog, he was home, and he was getting better.

Tom would continue to deal with extreme pain, which we attempted to control with narcotics such as Vicodin and Oxycodone for the pain, and Ativan for anxiety. He was also learning to deal with weakness on his right side, and moderate ataxia, or shaking, of his right arm, hand, and leg. Fortunately for Tom, he is left handed.

Salem, Oregon

The first year we were in Salem things took off on a quick and positive pace. My team at K/P was great, supportive, and driven for success. We had added fulfillment and direct mail services to augment our business, and we had grown 40% in that first year. We even managed to turn a profit, the first in Oregon operations in several years. But life and my focus were changing. Tom was energetic, fun, trouble and pretty much like any other normal kid. In 1999, I had focused on the community, my team, and current clients. I enrolled in Chemeketa Community College accounting classes in an effort to get a better handle on our business finances. I became involved with Willamette University, and the new President, Dr. Lee Pelton. Willamette University was one of our key clients. I focused on past clients, and deteriorating clients, as well as becoming deeply involved in the community.
I reached out to Dave, the owner of Lynx, a competitor. Dave is an extremely driven individual with a philosophy of hard work, and being involved at every level. Lynx is a very successful company, and Dave had the money to hire the staff he needed, and spend time on his ranch with his horses, but he and his wife worked the business, and took personal care of their customers. At any time you can find Dave working at his desk, out on the floor running a press, loading paper, or installing the latest press equipment. He worked hard, and demanded hard work and commitment from his staff.
With all that Dave had going on, he welcomed me into his facility and took time to give me a tour. He took me to lunch, and we discussed Salem, K/P, Lynx, the market, and his view on what I needed to do to be successful. He did not ask for anything, but willingly shared his time and experience.
During this time, I also joined the local Rotary Club and became the secretary for the board. I got involved in the annual Rotary auction, and procured a car for auctioning off at the event. That is where I met Jim.

Jim is a financial advisor and leader in the Salem community. He has a strong sense of community, and a desire to be productive in helping kids. It was this drive and leadership that drove Jim to start an annual fundraising event called "Hoopla". Hoopla is a three-on-three basketball tournament played in the summer on the streets of Salem. It is an open event that draws thousands, and raises hundreds of thousands of dollars for organizations that focus on youth athletic or activity programs in the Salem-Keizer, Oregon area. I was honored when Jim asked me to be part of the group that put together the inaugural event. Three of my team at K/P also joined me in playing in the tournament.

I joined the Salem Economic Development Corporation, attended lunch meetings, and hosted events. I was part of the gala committee, and worked to help Salem create an environment for growth. In 2000, though, all this began to change rapidly.

Now the guilt comes through. Did I work so hard and focus so much on things that I lost focus on my son? I had dreams of being a basketball coach for a team he would play on one day, but I did not play basketball with him enough.

Tom had always been a smart kid with lots of energy. Though he did little homework, his school grades were always exceptional, despite a frequent notation that he was sometimes disruptive in class. Tom often finished tests and assignments first, then wanted the attention of the other kids. He was challenged to sit still and read or do some other task. During the spring term of 2000, this began to change. He was still getting A's on his report card, but his behavior began to moderate. He was becoming quieter. He was also complaining of various ailments, mostly back aches and stomach aches. He would also have intense headaches at times, but when he relaxed they seemed to ease.

One spring evening, Tom began to scream in pain. His stomach was hurting. Beth and I took him to emergency, and had x-rays done of his abdomen. The images seemed to show possible gas build up, and he was given a laxative. Not long after, he was having extreme pain in his back, and again we went to the ER, and again, nothing definitive was shown. We began regular visits to a pediatrician, who scheduled an MRI for Tom's neck and back. Nothing out of the ordinary was shown on the images and he suggested Tom was just having growing pains. There were even stretch marks on Tom's back.

Back at Home

Now that we were back at home, and with my son fighting for his life, I lost focus on the business at K/P and the business began to slow. It was difficult to maintain the same level of dedication to the business. Back at home, Tom was in his room, still dealing with extreme head pain, needing follow up care, and his eyes were so sensitive to light that we had to cover all the windows in his room. No matter how hard I tried to complete my tasks at work, that is what they had become: tasks. I had lost my passion.

The words of Dr. Walker continued to haunt me. His first guess was that Tom's tumor was a fast growing ganglioglioma. The pathology told a different story, but Dr. Walker is a well-known, very experienced pediatric neurosurgeon. In my experience, when people like that make an observation it usually has a high degree of accuracy--something was wrong.

After surgery, Tom needed a MRI every month to check for recurrence and any possible complications that were not immediately visible. On the advice of Dr. Walker, we scheduled a follow up visit with Dr. Webe. Dr. Webe is a dedicated, kind, maternal woman with dark hair, a small stature, and a way of coming across as a friend. Her confidence, knowledge, and mannerisms left us no doubt that she knew what she was doing.

It was another warm and bright day at the end of September when we were making our way up from Salem to Legacy Hospital in Portland. Tom was doing better, but he was still in extreme pain. Some of the pain manifested as headaches, other pains came from more easily identifiable sources, such as the incision that had been made through the skin and muscles of his neck. We were going to see Dr. Webe again, and to get Tom's first follow up MRI.

Tom was doing better. He was healing and we had hope, but I could not get rid of the darkness. Everything I was doing was a task with a short time frame. Every thought I had was interrupted by the desire to know how Tom was doing, and by fear. My emotions were on edge and at times tears would just come to my eyes. My breathing would become labored and it would seem that the dark hole I was in was closing. So I focused on the moment and task at hand.

The trip to Legacy from Salem is pretty straight. You get on I-5 and head forty five miles north to Portland. There are three lanes in each direction of I-5 as you approach Wilsonville, a small town just south of Portland. Just north of Wilsonville is where I-405 takes off to the east and circles Portland. This was a weekday, and traffic was moving at a brisk pace of sixty miles per hour. We would be at the hospital on time, but I was still feeling scared, dark, and sick. As we were passing Wilsonville, I was surprised as rider on a green Kawasaki Ninja motorcycle passed at an extreme speed. I did not see the rider coming up from behind, and was startled by the passing of the bike between me and the car on my right. "Shit" escaped from my lips, and then the bike was out of sight. Two minutes later traffic came to a stop.

At first I thought that the rider of the motorcycle had crashed his bike ahead, but traffic was moving slowly, and the backup was well over two miles long. It took a half hour to travel past the off ramp and get to the scene of the accident, and then, there it was: the green Kawasaki Ninja on the right side of the freeway, and a covered body under a tractor-tailor, also on the right side of the road. Parts of the distinctive bright green fiberglass bike were spread out all over the lanes of the freeway. I was sick. I also ride a motorcycle, and wanted to help, but there was nothing I could do, and we needed to get Tom to the hospital.

Even laying on the cold table of the magnetic resonance imaging (MRI) machine was difficult for Tom. They had given him some pain medication, and Ativan, an antianxiety drug, but this was going to be tough. An MRI scanner is a device in which the patient lies inside a large, powerful magnet. An MRI provides good contrast between the different soft tissues of the body, which makes it especially useful in imaging the brain, and that's what we needed to see what was happening inside Tom's head. In order for the MRI to be effective and get good images, the patient needs to stay extremely still. Due to Tom's ataxia this was difficult, the pain made it worse, and the imaging took twenty minutes. To complicate the task, the MRI generates a series of loud noises ranging from the sound of a jack hammer to an irritating vibration-- it can be difficult to endure with a minor headache.

The MRI is a high powered magnet, so Tom needed to make sure he had removed all metal. I had worn sweats, and left my wallet, keys and everything else in a locker provided by the hospital so that I could be in the room with Tom. The technician put headphones over Tom's ears. Then the table, and Tom, slid into the large circular machine.

Even with the medications, the process was brutal for Tom. The technician talked to him through the speakers of the machine, and reminded him that he needed to be still. Some of the pictures were coming out blurred. He was patient with Tom, and Tom was brave, and tough. The technician stopped the machine and asked if it was too difficult, but Tom wanted it done, to leave, and not have to come back. After thirty minutes of this, the machine stopped, the technician came in, and the table Tom was lying on slid out. A nurse came in and gave Tom a shot of a solution to provide contrast in areas where the tumor or other possible lesions might be, and the process began again. It took almost an hour. Tom was crying and I was feeling worn out and sick, but we were done.

I felt weak, embarrassed, and foolish. Tom was the one going through the tests and the pain, and I was having a hard time holding it together. I could not let him see how I was feeling, he needed me to be tough, to tell him it was OK and how well he was doing-- not to breakdown, cry, and puke. I had to concentrate on every step. Each moment in time was all there was. It was dark, and about to become even more terrifying.

Thirty minutes after the MRI, we had an appointment with Dr. Webe. The appointments always started out the same. How was the pain? On a scale of one to ten, ten being the worst you have ever felt, how are you now? The answers were usually seven or eight, but that day it was a nine.

The next part of the examination had Tom try to walk heels to toe. He stumbled, not having the coordination or control of his right side to make this happen. He would have to practice. The rubber hammer with the triangular head would come out next, and his knees, heels, and elbows would be tapped on each side to gauge his reflexes. He hated the scope that the doctor used to see inside his eyes to look at the nerves--it increased the pain. The last test was to hold a finger in front of Tom and have him take the index finger on his left hand and touch it to his nose, to the doctor's finger, and then back to his nose as quickly as he could, while the doctor moved her finger several inches in different directions. The test was then repeated on the right side, and the difficulty Tom had controlling his hand was obvious.

We had been in the examination room for fifteen minutes with Dr. Webe when she put the MRI images on the lighted screen on the opposite end of the small room. As she began to talk, I could feel the room close in, spin, and the nausea build. She had copies of the last MRI from Children's Hospital in Utah and the one from earlier today. There were signs of enhancement, and tumor growth, and part of it was approaching what she termed the pons, the brainstem. Tom would need additional surgery soon.

I have vague memories of her suggesting that due to the original size of Tom's tumor and the nature of the emergency surgery, the abnormality of the shape of the brain due to the excessive pressure of fluid, and many other factors, this may just be a couple pieces of tumor that were missed. I don't remember any part of the day after that, or even how we all got home.

The void, that deep dark hole that feels like a cold burning of my soul, never quite goes away. This was thirteen years ago, and I still get dizzy, and the room spins as I think about those days, and I am not alone. After returning from Utah, my dad took my mom to the doctor to find out why she had been experiencing some bleeding and pain. They learned that my mom had uterine cancer and needed surgery. When I called my parents, they cried. My mom said "oh, God no!" and her reaction immediately went to postponing her own surgery and treatment. But my parents now had their own fight, one that was much worse, and would cause more anguish, than they could imagine. I had to take care of Tom, and dad had to take care of mom, and it would push dad and me to our extreme edges, mentally, emotionally, and physically.

Chapter 7 – With a Lot of Help from My Friends

One life I had a nightmare.
I dreamed I was walking along
The beach with my son.
Across the dark sky flashed scenes from our life.
For each scene, I noticed
Two sets of footprints in the sand,
One belonging to me and the other to my son.
When the last scene of our life flashed before me,
I looked back at the footprints in the sand.
I noticed that many times along the path of our life,
At the very lowest and saddest times in our life,
Our footprints disappeared into a mass of deeply trampled and displaced
sand.
I turned to my son and we knew
It was then that we were carried by the masses of family, friends and good
people.

Brian Yates

I was eighteen when Brian and I met at church. He had just returned from a mission and I was considering whether I should go on one. At 6'5", Brian is about an inch taller than I am and at the time he was in great shape. We would play basketball together, go to church, go to parties, and meet girls.

When missionaries return home and address the congregation, they almost always tell the same story: this was the best event of their lives. Brian was more honest with me and the other people he addressed. Like others, he related that this was the best thing he had ever done, and the experiences were amazing. He also added it was the toughest, most lonely, and hardest thing he had ever done. He talked about the desire to come home, discouragement, and about the dedication, and stubbornness that it took to complete the mission. It was this honesty that inspired me to complete a mission.

Brian and I lived for fun. We would work just enough to make money for the dates that weekend. We joined church groups and then led them down paths that were on the edge of acceptable behavior. We included everyone that wanted to join us. We raced our cars, and bought identical motorcycles. We raced the motorcycles down the street, at one point, close enough that he reached over and hit my kill switch.

While I was on my mission, Brian married Dorinda, and she became my friend as well. They moved to Utah, and after I married Pam, Brian gave me a job with the company he was working for in Orem, Utah. On one particularly cold, clear, winters night he also spent hours walking out to my car and pouring water over it. In the morning my car was a block of ice.

Brian was my friend, boss, and neighbor when Tom was born.

Richard Lancaster

I really don't know what I was thinking. Maybe it was because I was eager to make another sale, or maybe it just seemed reasonable at the time. It was the early 90's, and internet speed and bandwidths were limited at best--nothing like it is today. There was some commerce on the web, but only the most adventurous consumers would put their credit card information a web site. Who knew where it would go, and there were all kinds of warnings of account theft. If done in the US, production of a new software program took a month or more. To set up call centers and start a global program would take even longer. And yet, I told Pat we could do it in 10 days. The first vendor we partnered with had forgotten to pay their bills, shut everything off, and left me hanging. Pat worked for Microsoft, the largest customer that I had made this commitment to, and it was going south fast.

These were the conditions when I met Rich. Rich was the owner and President of Cobweb, a new ecommerce company that was stretching the edge of technology. My network manager had heard about Rich's company and thought I should talk with him. I called Rich on a Friday and he agreed to meet me on Saturday morning.

It was Saturday, and I decided I needed to spend time with Tom, who was 9, as well as getting this new business process started. The meeting should last no more than an hour, and I had a game Tom could play while he waited. Rich had just opened a new office in Issaquah, about a forty five minute drive from our home.

We arrived at Rich's new office and he was there, along with his 9 year old son Aaron. It was unexpected, but would work out great. The office was in a single level building and had new paint, a few desks with computers in front, a dart board on the wall and a computer at each desk. It was a very nice place. Rich turned on a computer game and we left the boys and went into a conference room to talk.

In the conference room I explained the program to Rich. We would produce a trial version of a program and take orders online for $4.95. His program would collect all the information for shipping and billing. I would contract with three call centers around the world that had internet access, and when they were called they would place the order on his site. However the orders came in, they were placed on one single site that he would operate. We would then collect those orders every day and ship them out. It seemed pretty simple to me, and we expected about 6,000 orders in a month's time.

Rich started by telling me about his company, and what they were doing with e-storefronts. He then began to educate me about the problems with my plan. He could collect the credit card information and send us a file with the address, but laws prevented him from charging the credit cards until after the product shipped. We would have to develop a system to confirm the shipping, charge the cards, account for returns, and a whole range of possible issues. This was a much bigger project than I had imagined, and we would need some support from the client.

We flew through the parameters of the program in what seemed like thirty or forty minutes, but when we looked at the clock it had been over three hours. We went to check on the boys, and as I walked out I saw Tom, eyes closed, back to the dart board, heaving a dart at the board. It hit the ceiling. I was horrified that Tom was putting holes in the walls, and ceiling, of Rich's new office. Rich blew it off. It was our fault, we left the kids with darts. No worries.

I trusted Rich and his partner Sean. This was the first of many programs we would do together, and in the first week it created 65,000 orders. (Guess our estimates were a bit off). We went to clients, openly explaining that I worked for Quebecor Integrated Media, and they were my vendor and partners with Cobweb. Both of our companies enjoyed great success.

It was not always roses and on-time deliveries. We had been awarded a very large program that was to be announced at Comdex, a global information technology event. The client had a short time line, and a kit that consisted of 9 CDs. We would get the last CD on Wednesday, the site would be live on Thursday, the announcement for the program would happen Saturday, and we were expecting 100,000 orders over three months. We would ship everything in the US via USPS 2 day express, and guarantee orders delivered three days after the order was placed. What could go wrong?

The client announced the program on Thursday but did not give us the final CD masters until Saturday afternoon. There were almost 200,000 orders placed on Thursday alone and the traffic crashed the site. By Tuesday people returned to the site to check their order and many placed a second order. We were critical, the site kept crashing due to high traffic, and the client, and their clients, were not happy.

Rich and I had an argument. Why were we not getting the orders, and why was the site down? I was standing in a cubicle raising my voice into the phone. Rich was yelling back that suggesting he just might turn the whole thing off if I didn't become more reasonable. When I was done I looked around and saw a group of people had stopped to see what the hell I was so intense about.

I met Rich later that day and we went out for lunch as we devised a plan to get the program back on track. Rich and I would work together on several programs, with different companies, and we became the closest of friends.

It was late September and Rich called. He was on his way down to visit. Salem is four hours by car from Issaquah, Rich drives it in three. He came down to talk, to visit a friend, and to offer some emotional support. This was the first time, but it would be far from the last. And it was only the beginning.

Mary Steinkert

Mary was wonderful, gruff, stubborn and very much like a mom. She worked with Brian and me as our administration manager. She did everything from greeting people at the door, to our creating our expense reports, to keeping us in line and providing counsel. She was amazing and she quickly became family.

In the summer of 1990, I was headed to Depoe Bay, Oregon for a week of fishing with my parents. I called and told them that I was bringing my admin assistant, and I could tell from the tone of his voice my dad was very concerned. He asked me if I thought it was a good idea and I gave an emphatic yes.

Mary and her husband Eric became close friends with all of our family. They went on a cruise with my parents, and joined the annual fishing trip on more than one occasion. And Mary loved Tom and Bug. When the kids would get rowdy she would tell them "if you don't settle down and behave I will beat you until your nose bleeds buttermilk."

Mary was at the hospital every day we were there. She loved Tom, Bug, me, my parents, Pam, Beth and cared for us all. Mary just loved.

Jeffery Demphile

Jeffery was the print plant manager the whole time I was at Quebecor. I got along very well with Jeffery. We joked, talked about clients, and he and his crew went to great lengths to assure my success with clients. I was part of his team and he was part of mine. When I left, he simply said "we are not done". I had no idea what he was talking about, and at the time, even he did not know the important role he would play in my life, that his actions would allow me to return to Washington and the care Tom so desperately needed.

Ian May

Ian worked in the corporate offices of Q-Media and was Jeffery's boss. Ian is a big guy, a Canadian with a good heart. With his dark hair and rough mannerisms, I thought Ian seemed more Australian than Canadian.

Ian did not really fit with Q-Media. At his core, Ian cared about people and thought that the business was there to support them. He and Jeffery had this in common, though neither of them could see it in the other, and neither of them fit the corporate culture of the company that had bought the facility and business they were working for from Quebecor. Jeffery and Ian gave me the support and opportunity that allowed me to provide Tom the medical care he needed.

Kevin Watson

I walked in while Kevin was talking with Alice, an accountant in our office. Her computer shut off and she was having difficulty getting it to turn on. "Have you tried the clapper?" Kevin asked. "These new models are equipped with a clapper to turn on and off, and sometimes a loud noise will shut them off."
Alice put her hands close to the monitor on her desk and clapped. Nothing happened, so she called again. Still nothing.
"Oh, this is a desk top and the CPU is under your desk." Kevin explained. "The clapper is in the CPU, you are just clapping at the monitor--you need to clap at the CPU." Alice crawled under her desk and had just clapped once when Steve, the IT manager, walked into her office and asked what was wrong. Alice told him that her computer shut off and she was trying to reset it with the clap.....
Alice turned red, Kevin got a huge grin and started laughing and I joined in. This was vintage Kevin.
Kevin's office was on the second floor of the building. His back wall was a large window that looked out over Tacoma. He kept a plaque propped up against the window, that when moved, displayed his picture with a speech cloud that stated, "I am wearing my wife's bra." The picture was attached to the outside of the window where Kevin could not get to it.
Kevin was the Purchasing Manager at Quebecor when I left and went to K/P. I recommended Kevin to take my position and dedicated a month to training him and introducing him to my contacts at Microsoft before I left. Kevin made a great Business Development Manager. Kevin also made a good friend.

It was November, 2000, and Tom was getting ready to have his second surgery. Over the next sixty days, these people would come together to create the events that would lead us to the best care for Tom, and the resources to keep us going through a storm that was just beginning.

Chapter 8 – 2000 NBA World Champions

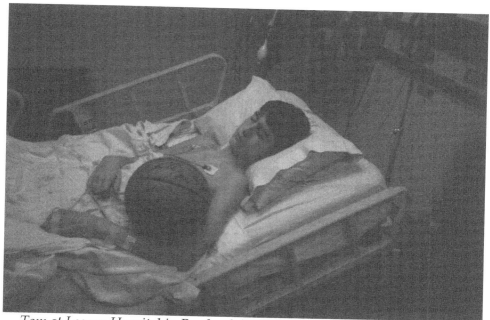

Tom at Legacy Hospital in Portland, he is recovering from his second brain tumor resection and holding his basketball that was signed by the Portland Trailblazers.

I was sick. Tom needed surgery again, on his brain. This was not supposed to happen. Tom was already hurting, he shook, he hardly left his room, and he should be starting school. I was already missing time at work, and when I was there every task seemed to be much more difficult than it should. Simple conversations would take effort and I did my best to assure no one noticed.

Tom had some time. The surgery would not be scheduled until mid-November. I was not sure if this was helpful, as we had time to prepare, or more difficult, as the monster had time to taunt us. What it did do was allow mom to have her surgery first, and even a few weeks to begin her recovery.

I sat in the hospital with Dad, Michele, and Steve as mom endured a hysterectomy to remove her cancer. Mom was more worried about Tom than her own surgery, I am sure it took some convincing that she needed the surgery and to take care of herself, so she could survive for Tom, and the rest of the family.

Anytime either mom or Tom was in surgery dad did not eat, instead he fasted, meditated, and prayed. Sometimes he prayed aloud with his family, asking God for health and strength for the patient and family, and skill and knowledge for the doctors and nurses. Most of his prayers were in silence.

Mom and dad had been married for over forty years; this had to be hard on him. His wife and partner was critically ill and his grandson was in a painful fight for his life. Dad was strong, he still amazes me and I wish I had his strength, focus on what is right, and fortitude.

Mom survived the surgery and a small piece of material was placed in her abdomen to emit radiation and kill any remaining cancer cells. Tom, Beth and I visited my mom in the hospital, Tom insisted he be able to go be there for his grandma, the way grandma had been there for him. But our time was limited, Tom was still weak, and most of our time was spent taking care of him and preparing for his next surgery.

Tom was still in pain but he still wanted an autograph. His second surgery was scheduled for November 13, just six days before his thirteenth birthday. He would spend his birthday in the hospital, so I made plans to take him to a Portland Trailblazers game just before his surgery.

The Trailblazers were doing well and most games were sold out. I bought tickets for the November 11 game against the Houston Rockets. I thought about Tom's desire to meet a player and get an autograph, so I called the Trailblazers office.

I wish I knew the name of the woman that I spoke with as I related the plight of my son. My emotional control was shot and my voice was shaky. I hated that the thought that my son was dying was forcing its way through my mind, wasn't it enough that he hurt so bad? I wasn't sure what I was doing, I did not even know if Tom could sit through a game.

The woman on the phone was kind and listed to my plea. She did not ask for proof, the diagnosis, or any further details, just asked me where our current seats were located. I told her we were in the third level but I could bring a wheel chair and take Tom anywhere. He could walk but he got tired quickly. She told me to please give those tickets to someone else, and she would have some better ones for me at will call. She told me to bring a new basketball, and remain in our seats after the game. A player would be giving an interview, and then we would be taken to meet him and get an autograph.

I gave my tickets to my sister. It was a Saturday, clear but cold. Tom was excited, this was the most lively I had seen him in a year. He wondered whose autograph he would get, and he held tight to his new basketball. We drove to Portland and parked at the stadium. We met my sister and Steve, and went to the will call window where the attendant presented us with center court seats, about fifteen rows up! As we got some food and made our way to our seats, my sister and Steve headed to the nose bleed section we had bought.

I bought Tom some ear plugs to block as much of the noise as possible. I had also bought some Bose noise canceling headphones, and he wore both. At times he took the headphones off but would place them back on after a short time. I monitored how he was doing; he was not always comfortable but he had no intention of leaving, not until his ball was signed.

The Blazers crushed the Rockets, 111 to 88. We were standing at times and I noticed that some of the times when the crowd when wild, Tom stayed sitting, and I sat with him. We stayed through the game and remained as the stadium emptied out.

While we were sitting, a chair, a stool really, was brought out and surrounded by cameras. Steve Smith, a guard with the Blazers, came over and sat in the chair to give an interview. While the interview was in progress a young man came over and sat by Tom and me. He introduced himself as one of the office staff and as Steve completed his interview he led us down to meet him and get Tom's ball signed.

At 6' 7" and 200 pounds Steve Smith is all muscle. He was soft spoken and mellow. We were introduced to Steve and he spoke to Tom for a moment and signed his ball. He spoke a few words to our escort, then turned to Tom, and asked him to come with him. Steve led Tom and me to the Portland Trailblazers locker room where we met each of the players; they shook Tom's hand and signed his ball.

Tom was excited. Scotty Pippin's hand was almost as big as Tom's entire body. Dale Davis spent several minutes talking directly to Tom, and talking about his family. Rasheed Wallace seemed upset and unhappy with the game, even though they crushed the Rockets, but still came over to wish Tom luck and sign his ball.

As we walked out of the stadium on that cold November night it seemed very warm. Tom kept repeating that this was the best night of his life. For the rest of the night he did not complain of a headache or neck pain, he kept looking at his ball, and talking about meeting celebrities, basketball stars, super stars, and how they had talked with him and signed his ball.

The ball is flat, the signatures are faded, but it is still one of the most precious items we own.

The Blazers lost to the Lakers in the first round of the playoffs that year, but to Tom and me, the following is a list of the 2000 NBA World Champions.

Greg Anthony
Stacey Augmon
Erick Barkly
Dale Davis
Gary Grant
Antonio Harvey
Shawn Kemp
Will Perdue
Scottie Pippin
Arvydas Sabonis
Detlef Schrempf
Steve Smith
Damon Stoudamire

Rod Strickland
Rasheed Wallace
Bonzi Wells

Thank you to the entire Portland Trailblazer organization and the night of relief and joy that you gave to my son and me.

Chapter 9 – The Nightmare Continues

Like all parents, I wanted to make sure Tom received the best care possible. I was scared. I started searching for information, reading everything I could, hoping to educate myself so I could make the best decisions possible. My biggest challenge back then was that I knew nothing about health care--how it worked, what made a hospital and its staff good, what challenges lay ahead. I didn't even know where to start, so I began by reading about pediatric brain tumors. I found articles like this description in Wikipedia:
"Any brain tumor is inherently serious and life-threatening because of its invasive and infiltrative character in the limited space of the intracranial cavity. However, brain tumors (even malignant ones) are not invariably fatal, especially lipomas which are inherently benign. Brain tumors or intracranial neoplasms can be cancerous (malignant) or non-cancerous (benign); however, the definitions of malignant or benign neoplasms differs from those commonly used in other types of cancerous or non-cancerous neoplasms in the body. Its threat level depends on the combination of factors like the type of tumor, its location, its size and its state of development. Because the brain is well protected by the skull, the early detection of a brain tumor occurs only when diagnostic tools are directed at the intracranial cavity. Usually detection occurs in advanced stages when the presence of the tumor has caused unexplained symptoms."
The more I read, the less I understood, and the more panicked I became. Pediatric brain tumors are rare, and the type of tumor Tom had makes up less that 2% of them. How would I make the best decisions for Tom? Where is the best care, the best hospital, and how would I know? My searches turned up information like this:
"Brain tumors in children are relatively rare, occurring in only five of every 100,000 children.
About 2,200 children and adolescents in the United States are diagnosed with a brain tumor each year.
Brain tumors are commonly treated with surgery and/or other therapies including chemotherapy and radiation.

All brain tumors are life-threatening, and many children and adolescents who have been diagnosed with one survive into adulthood. Many of them face physical, psychological, social and intellectual challenges related to their treatment, and require ongoing care to help with school and with skills they will use throughout adulthood."

All this knowledge kept the fear growing, and my head swimming. Tom was recovering quickly, but he still dealt with severe headaches. He was incredibly sensitive to light, so we covered all the windows in his room in order to keep it dark. He was lethargic due to the trauma and the side effects of the pain medications. We continued to visit an array of doctors and therapists to fight the pain and ataxia. It was a brutal time, and one of the people who really stepped up to the task of taking care of us was Tom's stepmom, Beth.

Beth and Tom had a difficult time connecting. A loving, touching, and physical person, for some reason, Beth had a tough time reaching out to Tom, giving him hugs or spending time talking with him. When I was gone, she would spend a great deal of time in our room, and Tom would be in another part of the house. However, she took over his schedule of doctor's appointments, organized his medications, communicated with the school, and worked with the insurance companies (over the years there would be several insurance companies involved).

I went to work and tried to keep the business moving forward. The few weeks we waited for Tom to have his second set of surgeries was excruciating and seemed to last forever. I wondered if it had been the best idea to wait for Tom's surgery. I wondered what damage was done, and if Tom would still be able to do the things normal kids do. Would he ever play sports, drive a car, or go on a date? I questioned if I had the ability to care for him. What about Bug? I did not feel like a very good father.

Head wounds bleed profusely. As it did the first time, Tom's second surgery lasted several hours, and he lost significant amounts of blood. There is always some risk with blood transfusions, and blood supplies continually go up and down. We were asked if we, and other family members, would like to give blood. We were also offered the ability to dedicate that blood to Tom, should he need it.

Interestingly enough Tom and I do not have compatible blood types; however he and Beth share the same blood type. Beth decided to donate blood for Tom, and we had that blood dedicated to his surgery. It became a small joke that Beth and Tom would become blood related.

Beth was supportive and made sure Tom had everything he needed. She did what she could to comfort me, and we both cried. When Tom was in his room sleeping, we would take turns checking on him, if nothing else, to make sure he was still breathing. When he was quiet, and between breaths, the seconds would become terrifying, fear would build that he would not wake up.

Then came the day of Tom's surgery. The weather was cool and the sky grey with low hanging clouds. At times during the drive there was a heavy mist, but it was not quite raining. It was a very typical Portland day. Tom was not allowed to eat the night before, or that morning. None of us ate; we just got up early and left for the hospital at 6:30 am in order to arrive by 8:00 am.

We arrived in the same red GMC Jimmy that had taken us to the hospital in Salt Lake. Going in through the hospital doors was like walking through heavy water. Each step took effort and each step added fear and anxiety. Tom was calm but quiet. We met my parents, sister, and her family and we started the process of tests and waiting.

We began the day in a small room where they were preparing Tom for surgery. As he had done upon his arrival in Salt Lake City, my father gave a blessing that morning, asking for strength for Tom, skilled and guided hands for the surgeons, and peace for us all. There was not much I could do for Tom; it was now up to Dr. Webe and her team.

Dr. Webe was using a new technology that was available due to advances in computer processing technology and imaging. Tom lay on a table, and what looked like a scaffold was built over his head. Then Tom, with the apparatus over his head, was subjected to another MRI. The placement of the scaffold and the MRI created a closer three dimensional image of his brain and tumor. This would allow for more precise surgery.

Once Tom was taken out of the MRI, he was placed in a surgery preparation room where we waited for almost an hour. During that time Tom was hooked up to IVs, and the top and back of his head was shaved. An iodine-based solution was placed where he had been shaved, to prevent bacterial infections during the surgery. His skin took on an eerie, orangeish-yellow glow.

The anesthesiologist came into the room and introduced himself. He talked to me to get permissions while the nurse gave me documents to sign. He talked to Tom, to let him know what was happening and give him comfort. Tom, never afraid to talk with anyone, engaged the doctor and asked him if he knew the difference between a zebra and an a-bra? "A zebra is 26 sizes bigger than an a-bra" --Tom always enjoyed having a new audience.

This surgery really was not a new event to me; it was a continuation of the first rush to emergency. The hollowness I felt had not let up. The fears were the same. Would Tom survive the surgery? Would he be able to walk? Would he still be Tom? Would he be confined to a wheelchair? The worst thoughts went through my mind, some that I am not willing to admit or explore even twelve years later. During the surgery, a nurse and resident doctor took turns emerging to give us updates on Tom's condition. All was going well. After several hours, Dr. Webe came out. Tom was in the recovery room, and it would take some time for him to come out of the anesthesia. The surgery went well and the tumor was removed. The pathology confirmed that it was a pilocytic astrocytoma, but she wanted to be sure.

Again, there was a question between what the doctors observed and what the pathology reported. To be thorough, Dr. Webe sent a sample of the tumor material to John Hopkins Hospital in Maryland, which she described as the best in pathology. After a few days, the report came back and confirmed the nature of the tumor.

After the doctor left, we began to wait for Tom to get into ICU. While we were waiting, a nurse came out and asked if I would come into the recovery room. Tom was extremely agitated and calling for me, they were having difficulty calming him. As I walked into the room he was screaming.

I went to the bed and did my best to comfort Tom. He calmed, but he was hurting, anxious, crying, and scared. Coming out of anesthesia is rough on everyone. You are in a state of knowing and yet not knowing. Dreams become reality, and you say things that would not leave your mouth at any other time. It is a brutal experience for an adult, it is excruciating for a scared kid.

As Tom calmed, he was moved to ICU where the healing would begin. ICU is where he was forced to move for the first time, and take his first steps. ICU is where his family was allowed to see him, hold his hand, kiss his cheek, and give him love. It was now after 5:00 PM and my dad gave another prayer.

Tom had trouble getting his legs to move again. The trauma to the cerebellum was severe and his control of his legs--especially his right leg--was hard. For the second time in three months, we started the dance. Tom would put his arms around my neck, I would hold on to him, he would place his feet on top of my feet and we would begin to walk. We would do this for a few days before he was able to put weight on his legs and take his first steps.

It was just a couple days after the surgery. I had not been outside and the shades to the windows stayed closed, so nothing really changed. Day and night were delineated by visitors, nurses, and activity in the halls. It was slower in the halls and somewhat quieter at night, though it was never really quiet for more than several minutes at a time. Monitors were continually going off, signaling low oxygen levels, drained IV bags, heart rate changes, and quite often, just a kink in a line. This time, Tom was hurting and the nurse had come in to give him pain medications.

The pain medications were the same ones he had been taking before the second surgery, a combination of morphine and codeine. But this time, his reaction was different. While in the hospital, the medication was being administered through his IV, directly into his blood stream. The nurse used an alcohol pad to clean the surface of the IV tube where the injection was made. She then injected the medication into the port, follow it up with a larger injection of saline solution to flush the medication into his system, and the medicine was on its way for immediate effect. On other occasions, the medication caused a cool feeling, maybe some slight discomfort, and then be followed by an easing of the pain. On those other occasions, as the medication worked its way through his system, Tom would inevitably fall into a deep sleep. This time he had a reaction.

As the medications worked their way into Tom, his veins began to protrude and redden. His arm immediately swelled and he screamed in pain. His heart rate escalated, he breathing became labored and his temperature soared. He was having an allergic reaction to one of the medications.

I don't know if an alarm was hit, if the nurse called for help, or if Tom's screams brought in other nurses and doctors. I do know that there was a flurry of activity and people. Benadryl was ordered and administered as quickly as possible, but even as it worked, Tom was fighting extreme anxiety. After what seemed like hours, but was really only several minutes, Tom was given Ativan, an anti-anxiety medication. He finally calmed and went to sleep. I sat next to him and watched him breathe, listened to the constant low beep of the heart monitor, and kept an eye on everything I could to assure he was ok.

As the days went by, Tom continued to gain strength. Friends from my work came and visited him; one guy brought him some more movies and a Playboy that had been bound into a Sports Illustrated cover. The Playboy embarrassed Tom and he gave it to Beth to dispose of. The one thing that was consistent, that each family member and some friends learned to bring with each visit, was a Slurpee.

We were all thankful when Tom was able to come home for the holidays. He even ate some turkey—washed down with a Slurpee, of course.

Chapter 10 – Off to Seattle

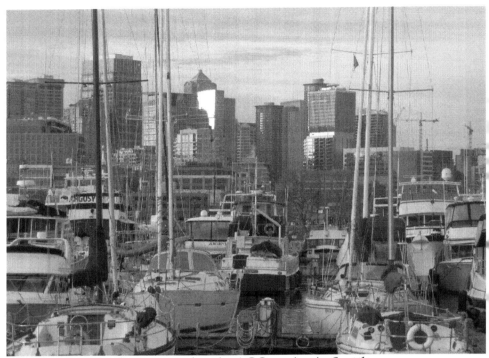

The view from our boat, moored at the AGC marina in Seattle, Washington.

Prior to taking over the facility in Oregon, I had worked for several years at Quebecor Integrated Media in Fife, Washington. One day after Tom's second surgery, I had a meeting at K/P's Seattle office that would take me past my old office at Quebecor, which was now called Q-Media. I stopped in to see the people that I had worked with, many of whom were also good friends.

Jeffery, who had been the print supervisor, was now the General Manager for the Q-Media facilities in the US, which included Seattle and Boston. My first visit was with Kevin, who was always wearing a grin and looking for solutions. Kevin and I had a few greatly needed laughs and shared a few memories, then we walked over to Jeffery's office.

Jeffery's office was on the second floor of the two story building. It was a large office with a big desk and leather couch. There were large windows facing north and more facing west, letting in a significant amount of light. The wooden desk was cherry, with deep reddish brown tones. The office was too big and ostentatious for Jeffery. His personality is caring, even-tempered, and egalitarian, not driven by ego, status, or authority.

While I was at Q-Media that day, Jeffery talked to me about the support I might need. He told me that I would be welcome back to his team, and he would do what he could to support me. I had recently read a US News & World Report article that gave Boston Children's a top ranking among hospitals for brain tumors; I had found other news articles that supported that. Seattle Children's was also in the top of the rankings.

So I picked up the phone.

I called the number for Neurosurgery at Boston Children's, and Dr. Scott answered. I was amazed, but I had reached the right person to give me information. I told him our story and he asked me questions about our location, our family's location, and about our support network.

I spoke with Dr. Scott for almost an hour. I told him I had the opportunity to move anywhere, including Boston, for the care of my son. Dr. Scott reviewed my story, as well as the medical records from Children's Hospital in Salt Lake City, and then gave me his advice.

Dr. Scott told me he found Tom's story interesting and that he would get great care if we brought him to Boston. But he also told me that we would need all the support from our family that we could get, and that if it was his child, he would seek out Dr. Richard Ellenbogen at Seattle Children's Hospital.

The timing and the speed of what happened next were incredible. Dr. Ellenbogen agreed to take Tom as a patient in his direct care. Jeffery and Ian made it clear that they would support me. The message was unmistakable, "Take care of your son and then take care of your job. We will support what you need and where you need to go." I was amazed at the support they offered--no demands, no questions, just blind faith support. It still amazes me.

Tom was healing. We had a house to sell in Salem and a place to find in Washington. I began my job back with Jeffery, at what had become Q-Media, in January of 2001.

My parents own a 38' fifth wheel trailer they used for touring. They offered the trailer to me to use as a place to live while we sold our house in Salem. I searched online for a place close to the Q-Media facility in Fife, Washington, and found the Majestic Mobile Manor and RV Park. On the map, it was located alongside the Puyallup River, just a few miles from my office. I did not have time to check it out beforehand, I just reserved an RV space sight unseen. We hooked up the trailer, and on January 2, 2001, my father and I took off for my new temporary place of residence.

The Majestic Manor was not quite what I would describe as either majestic, or a manor. The mobile home part of the site contains mostly late 1960's and 1970's mobile homes. Though they are technically mobile, they are fairly permanent fixtures. The RV Park is a gravel parking lot in the back. But it was close to my office, and met my needs while we were selling the house and getting Tom's care transferred to Seattle.

Fife is 195 miles from where we lived in Salem. The trip is about three and a half hours. For the next few months I would leave Salem on Monday morning and return Friday night. Tom and Beth would stay with Charlie in Salem, unless Tom had a doctor appointment in Seattle. During those times, they would come with me and spend a few nights in the trailer.

For those few months, I survived mostly on bratwurst sausages, cereal, and peanut butter and jelly. I also started stocking beer in the refrigerator.

The nights were quiet and peaceful. I felt guilty that I was not with Tom and Beth, and that I had a small, quiet retreat. At times, Kevin would stop by for a beer and we would joke for a while. The entire team at Q-Media welcomed me back and was supportive. As odd as it seemed, life was regaining some semblance of normalcy.

When Beth and Tom did come up, Beth would spend time looking for a new home. She really enjoyed looking at homes; I just needed a place to live. Fife is about an hour from Children's hospital and we decided that it made more sense to live closer to my office than to the hospital. The reason was logistics. I would have to drive to my office every day, and we would only need to go to the hospital for treatments, and hopefully they would be limited.

Time passed and work was going well. Months went by and Tom was not able to shed his headaches. He was not able to attend much school, so the teachers sent most of his work home for him to complete. Beth worked with the school counselors and Tom was placed on a modified school plan, adapted to meet his special circumstances. In reality, Tom missed almost all of his 8th grade year.

With the help of Jeffery, Kevin and Ian, I was able to work and support my family. Jeffery knew my strengths, and assigned me to accounts that were struggling or lost. This included Hewlett Packard and Intel, and both accounts became successful. With the help of my friends, I was able to get Tom the care that he needed, and be in the place he needed to be.

Our home in Salem sold quickly, and soon we were all united and residing at Majestic Mobile Manor. Beth continued to look, but could not find the perfect home. Our agreement was for her to find a home within ten miles of my workplace. Then one day, she came back excited, but what she had found was not quite a house. It was a cement slab. We bought a home that was under construction in Milton, Washington, five miles from my office. It was in a new housing development, and it would require that we lived in the trailer through June.

Milton is a small town about thirty miles south of Seattle on I-5. It is located in a series of small towns connected to Tacoma, and most people in Seattle do not even know it exists. What separates Milton from Fife is a road sign, a similar sign that connects Milton to Edgewood on one side and Federal Way on the other. At Milton's edge is Wild Waves Water Park and Enchanted Village Amusement Park, which is what most people in the area would recognize.

Every month for the first three months, Tom endured another MRI to check the cavity of the surgery for new tumor growth. The tests always came back negative, but he was not able to be rid of the headaches. The MRI did show that there was still some encephalitis, excess fluid in the ventricles, and swelling. Dr. Ellenbogen recommended that the valve placed in the top of Tom's head be replaced with a programmable model that could be adjusted with a strong magnet. Tom would require surgery again.

Chapter 11 – Beth

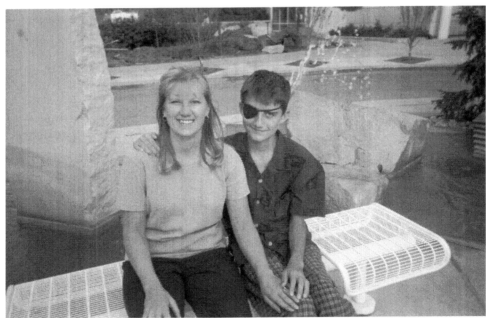

Tom and his stepmom Beth as we prepare to leave Children's in Salt Lake City.

Beth and I met while working for the same company in Orem, Utah. I worked in business development and sales and she worked in accounting. She was divorced, and I was going through a divorce, when she joined a group of friends and me for a water-skiing trip. I have always been addicted to being on the water, and water-skiing was a strong passion. My running and gym workouts were all focused on improving my water-skiing. I owned an 18 ½ foot Rinker open bow boat with a 210 horsepower engine. I loved that boat, the sun, the water, and the fun I found in all of it. By the time Tom and Bug were four they were on kneeboards and tubes.

Beth was beautiful, but so are many women. Though I noticed her appearance that was not what caught my attention. During that first water-skiing trip to Deer Creek Reservoir, I needed someone to back the boat down the ramp, and she volunteered. Backing a boat on a trailer behind a truck, down a long ramp can be challenging for anyone. Most people jackknife the trailer and have to make several attempts. Beth did not miss a step and backed the trailer in with ease.

The first time I asked Beth out, I went a bit extreme. Most people start with a drink, dinner, a movie, or even a nice play or party. As I think about it, we did go to a play on our first date--in New York. I had a trip I needed to make back east, and I asked Beth to join me. The original plan was for me to go to Boston. I extended that, and we started with a flight to Boston and drove down to Washington DC, stopping in Rhode Island, Connecticut, and New York along the way. Beth agreed to go, but the trip would be platonic. I agreed and was glad to have the company.

When we arrived in Boston on that first trip, it was late on a Monday. I went to the Dollar car rental counter, where I had reserved a vehicle for the trip. I had ordered a midsized car, and was informed that they were out of cars that size, and only had one car available that we could rent in Boston and return at the Airport in DC. So, we were upgraded to a new Cadillac.

It was after midnight when we arrived at the Marriot Residence Inn, located just outside of Boston. I am not sure how it started, neither one of us drank alcohol at the time, but we had a pillow fight and were roughhousing in the room. Beth went out to get some ice and was greeted by an unhappy guest from the next room, strongly suggesting we quiet down.

The trip was great fun, filled with new places, excitement, conversations, and tension. It was crazy to go on a date across the country with someone I hardly knew, and she had guts to go with me and expect that I would be kind and fun for a full week. There really was no safety valve. I admired her adventure and self-confidence, and we did have a great time.

Our relationship started with a lot of turbulence, dating, breaking up, and not knowing which direction we were going in. Over the next eighteen months, Beth must have broken up with me five times.

Over the next year I had moved to Ahwatukee, Arizona for several months and then to Loveland, Colorado. A month or so after moving to Ahwatukee, Beth's sister Tracy moved to Phoenix, about 10 miles away, and shortly after that, Beth moved down to join her. We started dating again, also resuming the cycle of breaking up. Ahwatukee is a small town just outside of Phoenix. Interstate 10 runs along the edge of town, and then heads south to Tucson. I was staying with my friend Michael. It was a crazy time filled with money, cars, and great parties. We would race from Ahwatukee to Tucson and back, checking to see if the trip was quicker in a Corvette or a Porsche 928. We would suddenly decide to take a trip to Las Vegas or up to a lake for water-skiing. We were living hard and fast and having a great time.

I was trying to forget my divorce, but I severely missed my kids. My life in Arizona was exciting and fun, but I needed to come back down and be more traditional in my career and life experiences. I took a job in Greeley, Colorado.

Greeley is a mid-sized town about an hour north of Denver. With a population of close to 100,000, it is a combination of agriculture based economy and academic--about half of the population is under 25. It is also close to a large sewage processing plant on one side of town and a massive cattle processing plant on the other--you could often tell which was the wind was blowing. Fortunately, it is also close to Loveland.

I bought a home in Loveland, Colorado at the base of the Big Thompson Canyon, which leads up to Estes Park and Rocky Mountain National Park. I missed Tom and Bug. Pam was also struggling and we decided to try and bring our family back together. Loveland is a great place for a family.

I spent as much time with Tom and Bug as I possibly could. However, the issues that caused Pam and me to split up had not changed, and it was not long until she headed back to Utah. For a short time I had Tom and Bug with me, and I enjoyed each minute, but that would not last long, and the Utah courts required that I return them to live with their mom.

I was working and living alone in Colorado, and I had not heard from Beth in several months. Then one afternoon I got a call from Beth, who was in Denver on a layover from a flight between Oregon and Colorado. She had left a message and I thought for a couple of days before I returned the call, but I did return the call.

We talked for a couple of times on the phone and it went well. We missed each other and wished each other well. I was done with our on again and off again relationship, but the words seemed to escape my mouth without thought. I had a trip I was making to Austin, Texas, would she like to join me for a couple of days? She said yes. I got to Austin the day before Beth, and I completed my business and visited my friends. The more I thought about it, the more I had decided that this would be the last time I would see Beth. She was great, in truth I did love her, but this was not a healthy relationship seeing each other, breaking up with no stability and I needed to find more time for Tom and Bug. Then I saw her at the airport.

I greeted her at the airport and we connected. There was a fire and deep connection that we had not experienced before and we had a great time exploring Austin. We talked about Colorado, the kids, Charlie and where we were going to head in life. We decided that the next weekend I would drive to Arizona, we would pack her things, and she would move to Colorado with me. It was just a few months later in April of 1994 that we were married. She was smart, she chose a day, April 4, 1994 so all I had to remember was two numbers, a 9 and a 4. 4/9/94. Later that year we moved to Tacoma, Washington for my job.

Beth would play a big part in my life and the life of Tom and Bug. Pam had an extremely difficult time with Tom, and we agreed that he would live with me. Tom loved Beth, but he was a young energetic boy, getting into things, making a mess, but never with malice and he tried hard to please everyone, including Beth. Though Beth had a difficult time connecting with Tom, she was very efficient at getting him what he needed and taking care of him. For years we would have difficult discussions about why she had such difficulty hugging him and feeling close. I still do not understand it. She was, and is, close with Bug, but she had challenges making a close, emotional connection with Tom. But despite all this, she was amazing at taking care of Tom and keeping track of his medical appointments, medicines, and educational needs. She managed the details and assured he had all the resources we could provide.

In 1998, I took over a small printing business and we moved from Tacoma to Salem, Oregon. Beth was having challenges with our relationship and our move, and I was clueless. My career and my life were going great. We had challenges, but they seemed to be minor. Tom was doing well in school, and financially, we were secure. We did not get to spend as much time with Bug as either of us wanted, in fact I had to fight Pam often for visitation, but we did have time and we were a family.

I did not realize how troubled Beth was with our relationship. I was not attending church with her--I never had. I had stopped being active in the Mormon Church before we met, just after I had moved to Utah in 1986. With parents and a family that was deeply involved with the church, my lack of attendance made Beth feel off. We had discussed it a bit, but it did not seem like a major issue. Then Beth reached out to someone else.

Beth and I contemplated a divorce. I wanted to stay together, work things out, she was not sure. Like many couples, we had a difficult time.

When couples or families are faced with major loss or medical issues, they often lose touch. It is a significant cause of divorce. The stresses are incredible, and Beth and Tom already had a tough time relating. On top of this, we already had a crack in our marriage. However, when Tom got sick, Beth changed her focus and we both focused on Tom and the challenges of keeping him alive and comfortable. The horrors of fighting cancer in our son brought us together with stronger bonds than I had imagined. She became key in our fight.

Beth stayed home with Tom, but had a desire to be productive as well, so she enrolled in school. Over the next two years she would complete classes on-line with Washington State University and earn her Bachelor's degree. Her first trip to the WSU campus in Pullman would be for graduation.

Chapter 12 – Aftershocks

The move to the new house in Milton was difficult at best. Tom was healing but he still had severe headaches. Most of his time was still spent in bed, even though his last surgery had been six months earlier. The windows to Tom's room were still covered, the light was excruciating to him. He had missed most of his eighth grade year at school, and now he was missing his summer vacation.

We would take Tom to see Dr. Ellenbogen, a Neurologist, an Oncologist, a pain specialist, and our family doctor. It seemed we would be going to a doctor several times each week.

Our family doctor was Jack. Jack is not really a doctor; he is a Physician's Assistant. Physician assistants, also known as PAs, practice medicine under the direction of physicians and surgeons. They are formally trained to examine patients, diagnose injuries and illnesses, and provide treatment. Physician assistants have a bachelor's degree. Then, they must complete an accredited educational program for physician assistants. That usually takes at least 2 years of full-time study and typically leads to a master's degree. Physician assistants are licensed and can prescribe most medications. To us, though, he is Dr. Jack.

We had seen Jack, and he had gotten to know Tom years before when we lived in Tacoma. Jack had served as a Navy Medical Corpsman. He had opened his own office in Fife, Washington, and I originally went to see him for a flu shot. He was easy to get an appointment with, and soon all of our general medical needs were under Jack's supervision. Jack liked kids and also served as the sports medicine professional for Fife High school. He also gave volunteer treatment for some underserved families. Jack is a good guy.

Jack cared about Tom and quickly became a key player in his treatment. We had all of Tom's medical records sent to Jack and he consulted with the specialists at Children's. He would see Tom and monitor his prescriptions, keep them filled, and watch for adverse effects. But with all the medicines, we could not get Tom's headaches to ease.

Dr. Ellenbogen scheduled another surgery for Tom. This one would take under an hour and replace the valve in Tom's shunt that regulated the fluid pressure in his head. There was no guarantee that this would work, and it is still a risky surgery, but Tom could not live in his room with the blinds closed for the rest of his life. Memories of the pain of surgery had not left Tom. The fears and horror of letting go of him as he was taken into surgery had not left me. I knew that we had come here because Dr. Ellenbogen and his team are the best. I knew Tom was in good hands, but I also know the risks, and I am deeply aware of the pain and challenges Tom faced with each surgery. This dark place we were in was not allowing in any light. My son was being tortured. If there is a god, why would he let a kid go through this? Everything happens for a reason? Are you kidding me? There is no good reason to torture my son. If there is a god he is a bastard, and I hate him. Those were my thoughts, and they were deep, and they would last.

Tom was scared; we all were. He was just thirteen and this would be the third time he was wheeled into a hospital for surgery, for a total of five surgeries on his brain. This was crazy, how many times can you open up a brain and still not destroy the person?

Some neighbors had heard about what we were experiencing, and came to talk with me. They were involved with the Make a Wish Foundation and believed that Tom would be accepted as a child in need of a wish. I know that the offer was given out of love, but I took it the wrong way. I thought that the Make a Wish Foundation granted wishes to dying kids, and Tom was not dying! Even if he was, I could not let anyone tell him that, were they crazy? I don't remember the exact words of the conversation but I doubt I was kind. I was uninformed, and I made a mistake that cost Tom a moment in time that would give him joy--moments that are extremely rare and valuable. I also drove away people that cared, and I never heard from them again.

The surgery was successful, but painful and stressful. Each trip to the hospital was getting tougher for Tom to deal with. The pain did not let up and the doctors would tell him he needed more surgery, and each time it hurt, and hurt bad. Then there came the medications, the depression, and the headaches.

Though his legs continued to work, the process of getting out of the hospital bed was still painful. Every move hurt. A sneeze or a cough would send Tom to tears and terror. The medications were increasing his anxiety, even as they would dull the pain.

We brought Tom home and the cycle continued. The light hurt his head and he could not find relief from the headaches. We would see all the doctors, they would search for a solution, we would try new medications and we would wait. After two months, though, Tom was able to leave his room and start moving towards a normal life. The new shunt and some of the medications began to help. Tom was still averaging a Slurpee a day. The cold drink was soothing and provided mental comfort as well. Along with the Slurpee, we would play video games. We had a Nintendo Play Station 2 and an X-Box. Microsoft had released the X-Box in November of 2000, just in time for the Christmas rush. Lines had formed and people had waited for hours to get one of the new gaming machines. It was almost impossible to find one--almost. We were still in Salem, and I was at Fred Meyers, walking out, when I saw a clerk waking in the electronics section of the store with two X-Box machines, and put them on a high shelf. I asked him why they were being put up there and he told me he did not know, it was just what he was told to do. I told him I wanted to buy one, he handed it to me, and Tom had an X-Box.

Tom and I played Halo, but our most common games were football and basketball. Even with ataxia Tom could master the game controllers much better than me. With Halo we would team up to beat the game, or he would laugh as he slaughtered me with ease. With the sports games, I had a fighting chance. He could still master the controls, but I had the knowledge of the games, and I would use that as long as I could. During this time, he also became obsessed at beating me at chess. He claims that he finally beat me, even with only half his brain left, and I continue to deny it.

Tom began to attend school on a modified schedule. Beth worked with the school to develop a program with the best possible approach to educating Tom. He would go to school part time and we would hire a personal tutor that came over three times a week. Beth would also work with him on his assignments and education.

My stress level was high, and I continued to run to relieve the stress. September of 2001 was an intense time for me. During his time in the hospital in Salt Lake City, Tom and I talked about many things. We talked about the future and what we would do together when he got well. We talked about running a marathon together and he drew me a picture. The picture was a stick drawing of a man and a boy crossing the finish line of a marathon. I ran nearly every day to relieve stress and to clear my mind. I was averaging eight to ten miles a day, and in September of 2001, Tom and Beth came with me to Portland where I ran my first marathon. Tom's stick figure drawing had been transferred onto a white cotton t-shirt with a statue of liberty on the front. This shirt was not exactly the ideal material for long distance running—in fact, it chafed my nipples until they bled profusely—but it was the only shirt I would even think of wearing. I have completed six marathons in that shirt, and happily bled through each one. It is a dream that one day Tom and I will complete a marathon together.

Chapter 13 - Challenges and Hope

2001 was a year of challenges, disasters, and healing. I was driving to work the day that the Twin Towers were taken down by terrorist planes. I wasn't sure what I was hearing, or if it was real. I arrived at my office, turned on my computer, and there it was. The disaster was unfolding across the media, from TV and radio to the internet. My world had changed, and now, with one extreme event, the world was changing too.

Tom was continuing to improve, and on September 30th he joined me at the starting line for the Portland Marathon. The run was difficult and it took me 4 hours and 23 minutes to complete. As I ran across the bridge to the finish line I could see Tom and Beth. My race had been symbolic of the fight for Tom's life and the dramatic changes that were going on around us. But the most important piece of all, in my world, was that Tom was healing. He was well enough that he wanted to make the trip to Portland and see me finish the race. We were in this together.

Beth and I continued the marathon of caring for Tom. Each month we went to the hospital for an MRI to check the wound in Tom's head, and to verify that the tumor was gone. Each month, it was the same long and quiet trip to the hospital. The night before we would all grow quiet, and though Beth and I tried to be positive and keep Tom's spirits lifted, it was always the same tough, quiet trip. Tom would be slow to get out of the car. He would be physically sick and depressed. His feet would shuffle and his shoulders would droop.

The appointments started with registration, and then directions to the basement for the MRI. We changed clothes to assure all metal was removed from our person, and filled out the check list: no metal, no piercing, no implants, and no recent metal work--nothing that would be damaged by the strong magnetic pull of the MRI. They would call Tom's name, and he and I would walk into a room with a big round machine, and a table stretching into a tunnel that echoed with memories of pain and terror. MRIs were always the first step to bad news and more surgery. And each trip we made, Tom would question if he would choose to have surgery again, even if he needed it. Was life worth the pain? There are some things worse than death, was this one?

The MRI process would take almost an hour. Two images were taken: one as he was, and another after he was injected with a contrast fluid. The contrast would highlight areas of tumor or other abnormalities. Tom's MRI almost always finished at 10:30, and the appointment with the doctor would be at 1:00. We would try and get lunch or find some other activity, but it would be difficult to eat, difficult to move, difficult to do anything but watch a television in the waiting room and fight fear.

In October of 2001, after he had endured another MRI, we received some great news. Tom could go three months until his next MRI-- he was free until January! As slowly as we walked into the hospital, his pace was now reversed, and it was difficult to keep up with Tom as we left the hospital. Leaving was always at a faster pace, on every trip to the hospital, no matter what the reason for the trip. Mom was healing from her surgery as well, though her recovery was slow, and Tom was becoming more active. He was still dealing with headaches, but they were easing enough for him to get out and even participate in school. The holidays were coming and life was good.

Friends at Work

At work, Jeffery had assigned me the HP account. Quebecor had a large book of business with HP and had even opened a staging facility in San Jose to support the business. However, both companies had ignored the changing markets and the rapid advancements in technology, so inventories were sharply overbuilt, and obsolete inventory was huge. The finger-pointing became aggressive, both companies took significant write-offs, and the San Jose facility was closed. When I took over the business, it had been reduced to a few thousand dollars a month. That is when I met Mark Bregante.

Mark was new in his procurement position and looking to make good decisions, develop relationships, and solve inventory and supply chain issues for the HP Desk Jet division. I spent a good deal of time with Mark discussing both our companies and our careers. We shared information and created programs that would benefit both of our companies, while allowing us to progress as well. Along the way, Mark and I became friends.

With Mark's help, I returned to success with Jeffery and his team, and, at least in part, justified the grace that he and Ian had showed in supporting my need to relocate. The medical bills for Tom were quickly piling up. Insurance had paid out nearly a million dollars in the first year, and the co-pays were significant. The associated costs, travel, education, rehabilitative services, and the large amount of rotating medications added up to staggering costs as well. We were fortunate to have savings and a great job to pay those costs. I could not help but wonder, what did other families do?

We traveled to Sandy, Oregon for the Thanksgiving weekend. Though Tom was still moving slowly and fighting headaches, he was home, healing, and doing relatively well. Mom was getting around too, and we all had a great deal to celebrate. My sister Michele cooked dinner at her home on the base of Mt. Hood and we were surrounded by family. My emotions were swirling, but mostly I was thankful that our family was together and surviving. I was grateful that my family was together. I was grateful for my friends and their help in my career. I was in awe of the people that had come together to keep us standing. With all this, I was also distressed at the continued pain that both my young son and my mom were enduring at the same time. Cancer--was there a connection between the two? Even then I knew that it was a foolish thought. I could not help but feel that this was some cruel joke, of which we were the brunt. I questioned my previous thoughts, growing up and going to church, teaching Christianity, and wondered if there was a God. There is no reason for this crap to happen--we did not ask for it. Tom, my 13 year old son, did nothing to cause or deserve this. No way.

Michele made a great turkey dinner with stuffing infused with cranberries and nuts. There were two long tables to fit the entire family, Tom, Beth, my parents, Michele and her five kids, Steve and four of his kids and a couple spouses. There was sparkling cider on each table, grape/apple, apple/peach and sparkling apple. Their fare included sweet potatoes, a bean casserole, mom's homemade rolls and everyone's favorite --mashed potatoes and gravy.

My sister is not especially religious; I am not sure when was the last time she went to any church, or if she has ever attended one with Steve. However, each time we have a Thanksgiving or Christmas dinner at her home, she begins the meal by asking our father to give a prayer. I do this when we celebrate a holiday at my home as well. We do it out of respect for our parents, out of tradition, out of hope. It is just about the only time during the celebration where everyone is quiet.

Between the kitchen and the dining room is a chest high bar with a marble top. The bar is eight feet in length and provides a separation between the dining room, living room and kitchen. On the evening of holiday dinners, it is lined with cheese cake, a very chocolate desert, pies (at least one pumpkin) and a bread pudding with rum sauce that Tracy, one of Steve's sons, would bring. It did not matter how much was eaten for dinner, the deserts were mouthwatering and would not be denied. I would try at least three.

Our offices were closed for the week of Christmas, so we traveled to Oregon once again. We stayed with my parents, in the house my father built when I was twelve. The home is twenty six miles east of Portland, between Dodge Park, a small park along the Sandy River, and Roslyn Lake, a small lake fed by a dam further up the river. It sits on a small hill situated on a seven acre piece of land, with a barn that housed four horses when I was young. There is a long gravel road to the house. Along the entire upper floor of the west side of the house are eight foot high windows that look down over a couple of acres of blueberry bushes, the barn, and a large field. In the middle of the house, again on the west side, is a large rock fireplace. Its rock construction is four feet in width and eight feet deep and runs from the basement floor and through the vaulted ceiling. It contains three fire places, one in the basement, one upstairs facing the living room and one on the other side upstairs facing the dining room.

My parent's room is on the upper floor, across the hall from my old room where I slept as a kid. There are two additional rooms downstairs. Beth and I would sleep in a room down stairs, Bug stayed in the room next to ours and Tom stayed in my old room. Each night I would wake up a few times to check on Tom. I would start by listening, hoping to hear snoring. If I did not hear snoring I would put my ear to the door and wait, slowly opening the door, trying not to wake him if he was asleep, but intent to calm my fear that he was not breathing.

We celebrated Christmas at my parent's house. There was a Christmas tree that reached to the top of the sixteen foot ceiling. Each bough of the tree had at least one ornament, collected by my mom through the years. Though there are hundreds, seemingly more than a thousand, ornaments, mom knows where each one came from, and each one is important.

Christmas dinner at mom's place has every bit as much wonderful food as does a celebration and my sister's. However, if there is one difference, mom has more cookies, pastries, pies and cakes. She starts baking goodies just after Thanksgiving, storing, freezing and hiding sugar and chocolate-laden treats. Each year, she starts with an apology saying she really did not do the baking she usually does, so there is not really all that much.

This Christmas, my sister and all her kids were with us. Beth, Bug and Tom were there, and my grandmother was there as well. I don't remember how many of Steve's family had joined us but there was a house full, and there were presents. I had been feeling fun and bought a small present for everyone, twenty some gifts, all the same, all wrapped, and I insisted that they be the last thing opened. There were plenty of gifts that had been opened and I waited patiently until it was time for everyone to open my gift. There was torn gift wrap and opened boxes all across the floor as I handed everyone a wrapped cylinder about three inches around and six inches tall. Everyone could tell pretty easily that it was some sort of can. When everyone had a gift, I told everyone to open them at the same time. As my dad opened his package and loudly proclaimed "NOOOOO!" it was too late.

As the gift wrap came off the cans, and everyone recognized that they contained Silly String, the race was on to be first to fire a long aerosol string at the closest target—which was, of course, a family member seated nearby. It is amazing how much of the string each can holds, and yet, it was all dispensed within a few minutes. The living room and everything in it was covered. There was string on the furniture, the Christmas tree, the lamps, and to this day, I do not know how some got clear up to the ceiling. Though we would clean the greatest portion of it up that day, years later, there would still be remnants of that evening found. Every nook and crease in that room and some of them in adjoining rooms would contain pieces of brightly colored Silly String.

On New Year's Eve, Tom and Bug stayed with my parents while Michele, Steve, Beth and I attended a party at a hotel in Portland. There was champagne and music. Michele and Steve are excellent dancers; proficient in ballroom dance, they also have favorites in country, swing and west coast swing dancing. Beth and I did well, but could only try and keep up around those two.

As midnight approached, noise makers were handed out and a countdown began. My thoughts wandered between the terrible events of the year, the coming together of family and friends to deal with them, the success I was having at work, new friends, and a healing family. At the stroke of midnight, the nets hanging above the room released thousands of balloons that immediately became targets for hitting around the room, or stomping on and popping. It was 2002, and we were feeling the hope of a new and exciting year. We had beaten the disease and were headed into a year of healing, health and hope.

Chapter 14 - A Crazy Year

Beth and I started 2002 off with a bit of over-the-top craziness. It was New Year's Day and the weather was cold, in the mid-30s, and cloudy. A breeze made it feel even colder. We had been up late drinking and celebrating, and yet, the next morning, it still seemed like a good idea to go water-skiing on Lake Sammamish, just east of Seattle.

While we were out the lake, our thoughts were of laughing, concentrating on water-skiing in adverse conditions, our friends, and having fun. In that brief moment, the weight of the past two years seemed to lift. Two years--wow. Those were a tough two years. We had hit an incredibly rough time, but it felt like we were finally headed back to the top. Tom was healing, though still dealing with headaches, Beth and I were doing well, my career was back on track, and 2002 looked like it was the start of great things. The big focus now was Tom's headaches and his education. We were making dozens of trips to Seattle Children's hospital and see a wide range of doctors, but the key doctors now included Dr. Ellenbogen to follow up on Tom's surgery and tumor, and the neurology department led by Dr. N.

There was a challenge with the medications that were being prescribed to Tom. Jack was consulting with the pain clinic, neurology was prescribing drugs that included antidepressants to help the headaches, Dr. Ellenbogen was prescribing medications to combat the pain of surgery, and we were getting worried about the possibility of drug interactions. Beth was keeping a record of each medication as well as a history of each time Tom had a headache, the exact time he took any medication and the results. We would share this with each doctor. We also met Kory.

Kory is a Physician's Assistant who works with Dr. Ellenbogen's group. Kory cared for Tom and our family and was extremely responsive when we reached out to her. I explained my concerns to Kory and we came up with a plan that she would personally review each medication and prescription that Tom was given, regardless of who prescribed it. She would also see Tom and help us find alternative solutions, exercises, therapy and healthy nutrition that would help him in his recovery. Kory would fill this role and guide us for the next several years.

Time was going by and life was slowly settling down. My job was going well, our new home was great, our neighbors were awesome, and for the most part we were happy. The challenge that remained was Tom's headaches. He was still having significant pain and sensitivity to light. It was Dr. Ellenbogen that came up with a solution that was radical, but might work. Unfortunately, it involved more surgery.

The critical danger stemming from the initial tumor was the buildup of fluid in the ventricles of Tom's brain. The resulting damage and the surgeries meant that a shunt was required to allow the brain fluids to drain from the ventricles located in the middle of his brain, down through his scalp, neck, and chest, and into his abdomen. On the top of his scalp is a valve that regulates the flow, and resulting pressure, of the drain. Dr. Ellenbogen would remove that valve, which had a fixed pressure setting, and replace it with a programmable valve that would be set to Tom's specific needs and comfort level.

This was a relatively short surgery, but still dealt with the brain and had significant risks. We talked about it with Tom, searched our souls, and decided to proceed. We had moved to Seattle to have Dr. Ellenbogen's experience. And Tom could not go through life living in a dark room.

A year and a half had passed since that first intense trip to the hospital in Salt Lake City, and the dramatic changes it brought into all of our lives. We had survived, and with the help of our friends, so many things were actually going well. Work with Q was expanding, I had become friends with Mark from HP and we were adding to the success of both of our companies. I had run two marathons, we had moved into a great home in Milton, and Tom was alive and seemed to have little damage to his cognitive skills. Yet with all the good news, my world was still dark.

Though the sensation is no longer with me, I can still remember vividly the feelings of darkness I could not shake. Darkness--I wish I had a better description, but that is what it was. Before Tom's illness, I was a forward thinker, a planner, always reaching for tomorrow, throughout my career, and life. Now I focused on tasks, what I had to do that day. I kept my calendar updated, scheduled meetings, and produced the work I needed to get out, but I had no ability to visualize if any of it would come to pass. I did not have conviction that tomorrow would come at all. It was difficult to hope.

Yet here we were, back in the hospital waiting for Tom to get out of surgery. The wait seemed like it took days. The clock barely moved. Was there something wrong with it? I watched the second hand on the clock and compared it to the hands on my watch. They both moved slowly and in unison.

Dark thoughts and fears rushed into my head faster than I could push them out. Meditation, prayer, reading, and talking with family did not work. The paranoia would not be denied. What if Tom did not wake up this time? What if he lost his ability to walk, talk, or think? He is 14, would he ever get the chance to kiss a girl, or drive a car? What if he never got control of his headaches? I tried to push out the fears but they would not go and they nauseated me.

After an hour a nurse came out to tell us Tom was in recovery, he did well and that the doctor would be out in a few minutes to talk with us. A little while later Dr. Ellenbogen came out.

The surgery did go well and Tom weathered it well. As soon as he was out of recovery, he was brought into ICU where we could see him. Coming out of anesthesia is difficult and unpredictable, and the policy is to keep parents out of recovery as the event can be scary. Tom had already been though several surgeries and had experienced the pain associated with the hospital as a young child. His anxiety level was high and his actions in recovery showed his fear. The nurse asked me to come back. Tom was yelling for me and he would not calm down, even with medications.

I heard Tom screaming as the recovery room door opened. "I want my dad! It hurts. Where is my dad?"

I walked over to Tom's bed and touched his hand and shoulder. I told him I was there and it would be OK, he needed to breathe. Please try to relax and breathe. It would take another fifteen minutes to calm him. It was brutal how he would fight the pain medications, refuse to sleep, and just become more agitated. Tom leaned on me and I leaned on Beth and my parents. It was exhausting.

The recovery for the valve replacement was much quicker than Tom's other surgeries. He was only in the hospital a couple of days before we brought him back home. At home, the recovery continued with extreme head pain, blacked out windows, and lots of sleep. It would be a few months before he got much relief.

Peace Takes Different Forms

Tom continued to recover, work was going well, but we were all stressed and exhausted. We needed a vacation, a quiet and peaceful place to relax. I thought about the beach and started to search the internet for vacation rentals. I had been to Newport, Oregon and loved the small beach town. I really loved the few times business trips allowed me to visit Newport, Rhode Island, where I had seen my first blue lobster. Newport Beach, California is bigger, but it is also a great place. My reasoning suggested that the beach at Newport, Washington would be a great place too. The problem came when I learned that Newport, Washington was not at the coast at all, but in the far northeast corner of the state, about as far away from the ocean as you can get.

Not yet realizing this, I clicked on an advertisement for Panhandle Lake Resort. The website showed a small private fishing lake with a seventeen hundred square foot home built on the shore. Though it was not close to the ocean, it did seem to be exactly what we were looking for. We did not expect to find a place that has wonders and beauties that cannot be described in words. Perhaps if I was Ernest Hemmingway, or James Michener I could some close, but I don't believe that even they could capture what exists in this piece of heaven on earth.

I traded e-mails with Mike Johnson, the owner of the property, and we received directions on how to get there. I told Mike about Tom, and our quest to find a place we would enjoy, and yet find peace. He gave me a little more description of what we would find and assured me that it would be very quiet, private, secluded and peaceful. Try as he may, he was not able to describe the beauty of it and how healing it would be for us all, especially Tom.

We scheduled our vacation for mid-June, just after school was out for the kids. We packed our GMC Jimmy and headed out on the six hour drive. We got onto Interstate 90 and headed east over the Cascade Mountains that still had white caps of snow and ice, past Vantage, Washington, where the freeway crosses the Columbia River and a herd of wild horses cast from bronze watches over the gorge from the highest hill on the east side. We continued to drive to Spokane where we turned north towards Newport.

Just north of Spokane, the terrain changes from an arid landscape littered with sage brush to green grass meadows surrounded by pine trees. In just a few short miles we started climbing into lush green mountains. Thirty miles north of Spokane we turned off the main highway onto North Diamond Lake Road and then took another turn into what is now a KOA campground. We followed the instructions that took us through the campground and the road turned to gravel and dust. One quarter mile past the campground we came to a gate made of five inch steel pipe across the road, opened the gate, and drove into Panhandle Retreat.

The modest beige house with a red metal roof looked new, and was more like a nice home than a cabin. The north side of the house had large windows and a sliding patio door looking out over green pine trees surrounding a beautiful, blue lake, with no other homes or people in sight.

There is a television in the house that we quickly unplugged, it is the only item that really seemed out of place. There was a note on the counter from Mike saying that we would not likely see him, though he would come by and empty the trash twice during the week we would be there, and a bill for the modest cost to rent the resort, which turned out to cost less than a nice hotel in Seattle.

There is a small boat dock with two row boats for fishing, one boat is fitted with a small electric motor. As we walked to the dock to check it out, we saw turtles everywhere. There were bull frogs croaking loudly at night, and deer would wander by from time to time. We were 2800 feet above the sea level that we had originally searched for, and we found the most amazing vacation spot I could have hoped for.

After unpacking I took Tom out fishing and we immediately began to catch large trout. We caught rainbow, cutthroat and brook trout, all of them large, and beautiful. When I had my fill of fishing Tom asked to stay out, and he spent hours more catching fish and releasing them. Later he would come in, and then immediately leave with his little sister to catch turtles and frogs. At night we built a fire in the pit between the house and the lake and roasted marshmallows, gazed at the night sky, sparkling with billions of stars undiffused by city lights, and listened to the songs of coyotes and frogs.

We had found our place of peace, and Tom had found a place where he could enjoy life and put some of the pain from his mind. Panhandle Lake became our place for healing. We have returned several times, and we plan on returning as many times as possible.

The Healing of Taekwondo, if only for a Minute

I had experienced many shocking events and thoughts over the past two years, but despite everything we had been through, I was not prepared for what was next. I thought he was crazy. There was no way he should do this, but Tom was focused on wanting to take taekwondo.

There was a taekwondo school in Edgewood, just a mile from our home in Milton that Tom wanted to attend. Beth supported the idea. I thought they were crazy; he had a hole in his head, a literal hole. Sta'rosa Taekwondo was calling.

We agreed to talk with Dr. Ellenbogen about the idea of taekwondo and Tom taking part, even potentially sparring. I expected Dr. Ellenbogen to help Tom understand that this would not be a good idea, and warn him of the many dangers, especially in a studio that focused on sparring. I felt sick, like a rock hit me in the gut, as he instead told Tom that he would be OK. Our trusted specialist told Tom to always wear a protective helmet, and to understand that when most people got hit in the head it hurt, for him, it would REALLY hurt, but assured him that the exercise and focus would do him good. So Tom started taekwondo lessons.

We agreed that if Tom started the classes he would go at least 4 days a week for no less than six months. Secretly I was hoping that he would not agree to these conditions, but he was committed. At first it was difficult to watch. The class started out with basic exercises and Tom as extremely weak. He had to do pushups from his knees and he could only do a few sit ups, but he kept going. Within four months he was keeping up with the rest of the class, as they started with 100 pushups and 300 crunches.

The summer had come and gone. We had spent time waterskiing and camping. Tom still hurt but was becoming more active and he was excelling in taekwondo--it was his long legs and arms, enabling him to outreach his opponents. At fourteen, he was 6' tall.

In September, I had the opportunity to take off with a group of five guys on a fishing trip, which we called the Bro Bash. We drove out to a campground just west of Port Angeles where we camped, played cards, and fished. In the evening as we got ready to play cards, my friends began to smoke marijuana. I was shocked and made some comments about it being illegal. I had not experienced pot in high school or college; now I was in my forties and my friends were getting high. As I made snide comments, they gave me grief about the bottle of Jagermeister that I had brought. One of my friends, Mark, kept referring to old movies and propaganda about smoking pot and laughing uncontrollably. I thought they were crazy, and was concerned about the legality of it and was pretty judgmental, but we had fun anyway. I had no idea of the importance that night would have in my life and in the care of my son.

As 2002 closed, we enjoyed a good holiday season surrounded by family and friends. Mom was doing well, and thankfully, neither she nor Tom were in the hospital. The darkness was still there, but there were good days, too, and we all smiled at times. But I was still scared, and 2003 was just around the corner, and I still awoke each night to check on Tom to be sure he was breathing.

Chapter 15 - American Cancer Society, the Beginning

David Allen walked into my office in Kirkland, Washington and told me he had heard that I had an incredible story. It was the fall of 2004, and he was wearing a dark suit, white shirt, and tie. David is not an especially tall man; standing a fit 5'9", he has a personality of a giant. He had introduced himself as a Director with the American Cancer Society, ACS. "Tell me about your boy," David said, as he took a seat.

David will tell you that I left him waiting for me for a long time; with a sly grin he says I did it to make him think I was important. In truth, I don't remember that at all. I do remember that he had learned of my story through Felicia, an account manager and contact of mine at Microsoft, our largest client.

I did not know much about the ACS at the time, though I recognized the name. I was immediately aware that David was working on raising money, getting major gifts from individuals and corporations. I was a little irritated by this--Tom was just healing from surgery and our own bills were flooding in. Between the stress at home, work, and the seventy minute drive to and from my office each day I was feeling tapped out. I sure did not feel like I had anything more to give, on the contrary, I could use some help. But I complied and told David our story.

David was starting a golf tournament, the North West Classic at the Broadmoor Golf Course, an exclusive, and elite course in downtown Seattle. Somewhere in our discussion that day he asked me if I would join the volunteer group that was leading the effort to get this going. Their goal was to charge $2000 a player and secure sponsorships in order to raise $200,000 for ACS programs. I told him I knew nothing about starting a golf tournament, golfed very little and really did not have much to offer. He said thanks and left. A few days later he returned with Marshall, a consultant from California who specialized in starting high end golf tournaments.

This really did nothing to change the fact that I had little resources to give, but I still ended up attending the first meetings of executives from various organizations to organize the tournament. Somehow I also agreed to field two teams, for a minimum of $12,000. Within a few months, David had come up with several crazy ideas, including dedicating the first tournament to Tom's story and having Tom and me give a presentation at the dinner and award ceremony. I had never done this before, but even then it was a compelling story and I was honored to tell it. Tom was only 14 but he would do well also.

I managed to pull two teams together from people I had worked with in the past. One of the teams was made up of me, a colleague from Germany and two from Ireland. I did not know much about golf etiquette but I knew that many people drank on the golf course, and it was a social event. I also knew that I wanted my guests to feel well taken care of and appreciated, so I added my own personal touch.

I did not spend much time gathering information about the ACS, cancers, the mission and the major messages that were driven home by the organization. So, I brought a gift for each member of my golf team that included a flask of fine scotch and three very nice Cuban cigars. The event photographer took a great picture of my team, each of us with our golf clubs and cigars.

As the event began, Tom was introduced and there was a small dedication. The day was clear and warm and the course was beautiful. Built in 1924, the large clubhouse is adorned with cherry floors, high ceilings, and intricate carvings. The rolling course, with tightly managed greens and long fairways, is reminiscent of the Irish courses and the visions of A. Vernon "Mac" McCann, who emigrated from Ireland in 1908 and became a leading golf course architect of the time.

Unfortunately Tom was not feeling well at all and was not able to attend or present at the end of the event, so it was just me. I told of the horror of being a parent with a young child fighting for his life, of the fear and feeling of utter darkness while waiting through surgery. I spoke of the feeling of loss of control, of seeing my son hurt beyond imagination and wishing nothing more than to take that pain. I spoke of being with Tom as he learned to walk again and of the mixed emotions of sorrow, pain as he hurt, and complete elation that he was indeed walking. That large room filled with people that had been drinking, laughing, playing golf and being very noisy, became as quiet as the bottom of the ocean.

The Next Event

David invited me to a Goodtimes Wine event, a social for people involved with the Goodtimes Wine Auction. The Auction raised money to send kids to Camp Goodtimes, a camp for kids with cancer and their siblings. I met several people there, including Suzanne Williams, a highly energetic woman who commanded attention, not only from her beauty, but from her forceful personality. She was another high level executive hosting the event in her large, beautiful home in the estates of Woodinville.
Beth and I decided to work with the Goodtimes Wine auction and I secured a couple of items for the auction and we attended the event, where I was asked to present Tom's story once again. It was an amazing black tie event at the Harbor Club in Bellevue, high in the tower and looking out over the city. As I spoke about Tom, his challenges, what we faced as parents, and how he had found the strength to walk again, return to school, and face the future that we all knew were full of challenges, the room was filled with emotion and tears. Right after the presentation the auctioneer asked for a general paddle raise for donations to fund college scholarships for kids with cancer. Along with our donation, the paddle raise netted over $25,000. I noticed that Suzanne made a $5,000 donation that night.

The Goodtimes wine auction was an incredible event. Beth and I became friends with David and his wife Katya. They had met at Washington State University, married, and had been living in Bellevue since. We later learned that the Goodtimes Wine Auction was the brain child of David and Katya and was started by the wine club they were involved with at the Harbor Club. David and Katya do not have kids but they had dedicated a great deal of their time and resources to supporting children in need.

I had no idea where this would lead, how important the ACS would become in our lives and how integrated I would be with the organization and other volunteers. As I write this ten years later I think of some of my closest friends, David, Katya, and Suzanne, that I met because David came into my office and asked me to tell him about my boy. We are still involved in Camp Goodtimes and in the continued adventures in Tom's fight with the effects of cancer.

Crazy Fun

It seems that the more intense and stressful my life events are, the more extreme, crazy things I need to do for fun in order to shake the pain out of my mind and calm my soul. It seems that Tom and I share that need.

2003 started much the same way that 2002 did. There was a light snow falling and after a night of celebration Beth and I went waterskiing with my friend Van on Lake Sammamish. Van and I had met at some event where we were drinking too much vodka and came up with an idea to water-ski on New Year's Day, regardless of the weather. After we each completed the first water-ski run of the year, we popped the cork on a bottle of champagne and toasted the New Year. We then loaded the boat on the trailer and headed for the hot tub where Anne joined us and we drank more champagne and thought about how crazy it was to go water-skiing in the snow.

The Fight for Healing

Jerry, Tom's taekwondo instructor and owner of the studio where he trained was marvelous. A former Olympic contender he stands about 5'9" and has a body that rips muscle. The focus of his studio was training for sparring, or controlled fighting in a tournament environment. Though the nature of the sport is violent there was no anger in the class. The shouts were to expel air from the body and produce great force and control, not sounds of intimidation or fear. Tom was back in school, Beth and I were enjoying life, and things were returning to normal. Tom's commitment to taekwondo was amazing, he was attending his class 5 to 6 days a week and sparring on a regular basis. Jerry is a great teacher with a balance of strong discipline, patience and care. He understood Tom and his limitations but he pushed him, and Tom responded by giving him his all.

I had the opportunity to hold the first board that Tom broke with a kick. And I had help, as it became two and three boards that he broke with kicks and hits. Tom was excelling, he was sparring, and he was winning. At times I would become emotional as I watched him work out and fit in with his class. Everyone respected Tom but no one cut him any slack or went easy on him, and that was just how he wanted it.

Tom was extremely excited when he came home to talk about the regional taekwondo tournament. Though Tom had never been in a tournament, Jerry had managed to let him be accepted into the regionals. At 15, Tom would spar with the 15 and 16-year-olds, and as a greenbelt he would spar with the green and blue belts. He would be sparring with kids older and more advanced than he was, and yet he was sure that he was going to win.

Tom made sure that he went to all his classes and worked hard. His favorites were axe kicks, roundhouses and sidekicks. He had long, powerful legs, and he knew how to use them. Jerry held strict discipline, and he made sure Tom knew all the rules, how to spar and how to work within the competition. Jerry taught Tom the patience, the courtesies, and how to stay aggressive and focused. Jerry taught Tom how to focus on his strengths and not give up.

In the days leading up to the tournament, I tried to caution Tom against being too cocky. After all, Tom had had multiple brain surgeries and had been sick for a long time. He had to learn how to walk twice and his last surgery was just over a year ago. I didn't think Tom would make it very far through the tournament, and I did try to soften the blow. Even with that I was very proud of him for his desire to get here, and just have his first fight. The tournament was just a couple weeks away and I was sweating it. We met at Sta'rosa studios early on the morning before the tournament began. There was a caravan of cars and trucks from Jerry's club that made the trek. All the participants were dressed in jeans and other comfortable clothes, and packing their sparring gear. At 10:00 in the morning we arrived at a school with a large gym, there must have been 300 people ready to fight.

Beth and I sat in the bleachers as Tom and his team met in a corner of the gym and prepared for the day. The brackets were posted on a wall. The gym was divided into six areas where matches were taking place, each with its outlined area and judges. Tom's first match came at 11:00 and was in a corner close to the bleachers where we could get a good view. We were nervous and hoped he would be OK.

Tom was matched up with a kid who was 16, a year older than Tom, and a blue belt, a grade higher than Tom. I was nervous that this would be a quick day. The two met in the center of the ring and received instructions from the referee. The match would be scored by clean, unblocked hits. Each round would last 3 minutes for a total of three rounds. Hits to the head, groin, kidneys or sweeps to the legs would not be allowed and if used would cause disqualification. The two fighters bowed and the match began. Tom was significantly taller than his opponent and had received exceptional training from Jerry, and it showed very quickly. His opponent scored the first point, but that was all he scored. Tom's long reach, legs, and training paid off and he won his first match. It was amazing and exciting. I could not believe it. A year ago he could hardly do a push up. Two years ago I was helping him learn to walk again. Now he had won his first match in a taekwondo tournament. Today was a great day, if he did not score another point, what he had accomplished was incredible. But he did score another point, and more victories.

Tom won his next two matches and was even more determined to win the tournament and a gold medal. He was fighting older, more experienced kids but having little trouble getting through the rounds. The excitement and adrenalin took over and he did not even notice any headache. The constant conditioning, 300 sit ups and 100 pushups before every class was paying off. The dedication to completing at least that many each night, outside of class, was showing. Tom was not tiring.

The Finals

Tom made it through the brackets to the final match. His opponent looked to be almost half his size. I did not know his age, he was a blue belt, but he was the least intimidating of the matches for the day. Again they met in the center. This time it was the only fight taking place. The judge gave instructions, they bowed, and the match began.

Tom's opponent came at Tom hard and Tom responded with a strong side kick that caught the contender in the center of the chest and took him off his feet. He hit the ground hard, his breath knocked out of him. Taekwondo is not like boxing, this was not the end of the match. The fight was stopped for a moment as the kid shook off the hit and returned to his feet.

Tom was feeling bad, he did not want to hurt anyone, it was just a hit, they had pads on and his kick was out of instinct. I could hear him tell Jerry that he did not mean to hit him and asked if he would be OK. Jerry assured him he was doing well and counseled Tom to concentrate.

The two fighters returned to facing off and no more hits were scored in that round. Both returned to their corners to receive instructions from their coaches. Two minutes later they returned to the center of the ring where the judge restarted the contest.

Tom's opponent and his coach had seen Tom's reach and power at the end of that reach. They realized that their strength was in close proximity and speed, and his opponent stuck with that. He charged Tom quickly and threw a fast combination of hits and kicks that Tom could not block. There was not a great deal of power in the hits, but that did not matter in the competition scoring, what mattered was they were clean and they hit the target. Tom suffered his first and only loss for the day.

At the end of the tournament there was a podium where each of the top three competitors from each group received a medal. Emotions ran through me as Jerry stood with Tom and placed the second place medal around his neck. I was so proud. Tom had won. In so many ways, against so many odds, Tom had won. He was on top of the world and he deserved it.

Chapter 16 – Really, at Forty?

This was great. Rich, Mark, Mike, JT, JW and Oscar met at my house early Thursday morning. We were headed up to the John Wayne campground just east of Port Angeles for a weekend of fishing and fun. We had tents, sleeping bags, enough food and beer for a month, cards to play poker at night, and I brought an ample supply of Jagermeister. I was also bringing my 19 foot Campion boat for fishing.

We took two cars, and the three hour drive to the campground was filled with discussions about business, politics, the state of the economy, and Rich's theories on how it was all manipulated by a shadow group of powerful businesses, and that the economy was going to crash.

There was no shortage of jabs taken at each other, all in fun, and all to get one leg up. This was going to be a weekend of guys competing, having fun, catching fish, bragging and just plain giving each other shit.

We got to the campground and set up our tents, and though it was late summer, it was summer in Washington, which meant we had rain and cool air. But even so we were having a good time. We set up the tents, built a large fire and cooked dinner.

After dinner, as we were getting ready to play poker, Rich pulled out some pot and started to roll a cigarette mixed with tobacco and pot. I was shocked, I had not seen pot since high school and these were businessmen in their forties. I told Rich I could not believe he was doing that and Tom agreed. I quickly realized that Tom agreed because he could not believe Rich would screw up good pot with tobacco. I soon learned that I was the only one there that did not smoke pot on these trips and I was going to take a ton of grief about being so uptight and drinking my Jagermeister.

Mark started the razzing by making a contorted face and saying, "yes Randy, we are all going to get high and laugh uncontrollably", after which he through back his head and laughed. That started a discussion about old movies from the sixties and seventies and how they portrayed pot as this terrible drug that melted your mind and took you into heroin and acid as a gateway drug.

I was anxious as they smoked on my new boat. No one had smoked on my boat before and I did not want to get any burns in my new seats. I was paranoid about cops, park officers, anyone that would bust us. I had no experience with this and my ignorance showed. I am sure I provided them with a great deal of entertainment.

We caught one salmon and cooked it the second night. We had long discussions on the use of marijuana compared to alcohol. They told me that it really relaxed you, gave you a peaceful buzz, unlike alcohol that just exacerbates your mood, and makes some people very aggressive and angry. They assured me that no one got into a fight because they were high, while there are millions of examples of people fighting, even shooting each other, when drinking. I had not smoked pot before and I was not going to start that night, but I learned a lot about it and had my first opportunity to observe people while they were stoned, and it was nothing like I had imagined.

We had a great trip and a great deal of fun. What amazed me the most after it was done was they still invited me to another poker game and to be part of their group. I had been the outsider, been the nervous one, and they were accepting and fun. I had no idea how important that was going to be.

The Weight of the World

Life was great. Tom was feeling better, my job was going well, Beth and I were having a great time and meeting new people, and it was early summer and just a month after Tom had earned his silver metal. Tom's follow up MRI and doctor's appointment was coming up, just a formality, and a time for Tom to show Dr. Ellenbogen his medal and tell him about the tournament.

Beth did not go with us to the MRI appointment. She had been to every other one but there really was no reason for her to attend this one. The MRI would last an hour, Tom and I would go have a burger and return in an hour to meet with Dr. Ellenbogen for 10 minutes and we would leave. We had been doing this for the past year.

Tom and I joked on the way up to Seattle Children's hospital. The sun was out and it was a good June day. The MRI was on time and went smoothly. We had lunch at Burger Master and talked about the tournament, what we should do for summer, waterskiing, and just general fun stuff. Our steps were light and Tom had a huge grin plastered on his face as we were led into the room where Dr. Ellenbogen would meet us, show us the MRI films, put Tom through a range of motion tests and tell us to come back next year. The nurse was taking Tom's blood pressure and Tom and I were arguing playfully about whether or not he was as tall as I am. When Dr. Ellenbogen walked into the room a weight followed him that was unmistakable. Before he said "guys, I have some tough news", I could feel my breathing become labored and see Tom's shoulders slump. Even the lights seemed to grey.

Dr. Ellenbogen put the films on the x-ray viewing board. He showed us where the tumor had been, the large cavity where it had been removed, and the places, not one place, but places, where the uncontrolled growth was returning. One of those places was against the brain stem.

He told us that he would need some time to study this some more, to talk with the radiologist and oncologist and come up with a plan. He could not do any more for us that day; his nurse would make an appointment for us to return.

Tom still told him about the tournament, how he had taken second place, and how hard he had worked. Dr. Ellenbogen was genuinely happy for Tom, but the dark cloud of the MRI results overshadowed everything.

The trip back home was quiet. Tom sank into his seat and stared out the window. I tried to catch the tears from coming out of my eyes, my voice cracking each time I tried to talk. The black hole had returned. No, it had never left; it had just hid for a moment and now covered everything.

Beth cried when we told her the news. There were a lot of questions and not much to say. We would have to wait until our next appointment. We called my parents. You could hear the air leave my father's lungs and the void build. My mom wept and said "that poor boy, hasn't he been through enough?" Whatever happened, they would all be there.

It was a week until the next appointment. It was a somber, grueling week. I thought back to that night in the tent when Tom had his seizure, and the next day when we learned he had a brain tumor and the surgeries started. The demon had returned, and this time he was giving us time to think about it, remember, and build fear. As the week passed we tried to do things that would be fun, tried to take our minds off the coming challenges, we tried to appreciate the moment, but it was difficult, impossible, for us to do. Tom was filled with fear as he told me "Dad, I can't do this again", and as tears welled in his eyes and fear built up in his voice, he finished, "it hurts so bad."

Every step, every day, became a challenge. I wondered what was worse, the shock of Tom's seizure and quick trip to surgery or the waiting, wondering what would be next. All of our moods were somber. Tom's headaches got worse and he spent more time in bed, all the time taking prescription pain medications to deal with it.

Decision

Tom, Beth and I walked into Children's Hospital in Seattle to meet with Dr. Ellenbogen. This appointment was different. We were not shown into an examination room or seen by a nurse. We were led to a conference room with a large wooded table and chairs on rollers. This was more like a business meeting than any medical appointment I have been to.

Dr. Ellenbogen came in with two other doctors, the Chief of Oncology and the Chief of Radiology for University of Washington Medical Center. We were introduced; they shook hands with all of us and asked Tom how he was doing. Tom's response was somber as he tried to add a little joke and said he was OK until he got here. Dr. Ellenbogen explained that the tumor Tom had was defined as a pilocytic astrocytoma. However, his tumor was not behaving like any pilocytic astrocytoma they had ever seen. The pathology had been checked in labs from Bethesda to Seattle and the results were the same. The doctors talked about what could be done: more surgery, radiation, trial chemo, or wait and see what happens. The Oncologist, Dr. Guyer, was somber and explained that while some tumors react to chemotherapy, the one Tom would have to endure had a likely result of damaging critical parts of his brain.

We talked about various radiation options being able to target specific cells, but Tom's tumor was spreading and there was not a way to assure that they would be able to destroy all the affected cells in this manner. They talked about removing the tumor one more time. All these were options, individually or in concert, but they all had one big additional challenge. The tumor was growing dangerously close, or even into the brain stem. If the stem was damaged Tom would die.

I felt hollow, I wanted to puke, and I was angry that Tom had to hear this. I could see the fear in Beth, feel her hand as it squeezed tightly around mine, and I watched Tom, a 15 year old kid, sit quietly, scared and hurting. Panic was setting in and I was losing rational thought. Was my son going to die a slow, tortured death? That is exactly what this was, physical and mental torture. How could he, how could we, survive this?

After listing to the options I asked Dr. Ellenbogen what the best course of action would be. His response shocked me. He told me "I don't know, it is really academic. You will have to decide."

ac•a•dem•ic [ak-uh-dem-ik]
adjective
1. of or pertaining to a college, academy, school, or other educational institution, especially one for higher education: academic requirements.
2. pertaining to areas of study that are not primarily vocational or applied, as the humanities or pure mathematics.
3. theoretical or hypothetical; not practical, realistic, or directly useful: an academic question; an academic discussion of a matter already decided.
4. learned or scholarly but lacking in worldliness, common sense, or practicality.

Theoretical or hypothetical; not practical, realistic, or directly useful? Lacking in common sense, or practicality? I was sitting with some of the world's foremost authorities on this and that is the best they could offer for my son's life?

The two other doctors left and I followed Dr. Ellenbogen outside the conference room. I was upset and I really do not remember exactly what I said or in what tone but the meaning was clear. I had moved my family to Seattle for him. He was the best pediatric neurosurgeon in the world and I moved my family here so he could save Tom. I am not an academic, I am not a doctor, and what would he do if it was his child? I needed his guidance. We needed his guidance.

Dr. Ellenbogen struggled; he weighed his training in medical ethics, his patient responsibility, his legal liability, the policies of the hospital and his love for Tom. Then he told me, "Randy, I would do everything I could to stop this now. I would remove as much of the tumor as we can and use conformal radiation to destroy what is left. "

Tom, Beth and I went home thinking about what we heard. We have a few days to think, meditate, pray, and talk to family about what we would do before we needed to make a decision. As we talked on the way home, Tom made the decision for us.

"Dad, I can't keep doing this. Let's have them do the surgery and the radiation and everything that they can one last time and hope it works. I am not afraid to die but this hurts and I just can't keep doing this anymore."

Again

One more time. One more time Tom was in surgery with his head split open from the crown to the base of his neck. One more time his brain had access to the outside air that it had never been meant to see. One more time pieces of flesh and brain matter were being removed in an attempt to save his life and ease his pain. And one more time we waited.

Beth, Tom and I arrived at the hospital together. My parents were there to meet us after making the four hour drive from their home in Oregon. We had almost gotten used to the process by now. We were call in from the waiting room and Tom got dressed into a hospital gown. He then lay down on a bed in the preparation area while we talked. Nurses and doctors came into talk with us for a minute. The anesthesiologist came in and introduced himself to Tom and asked if we had any questions. Soon Tom was taken to the operating room and we all moved to the waiting room.

The waiting was the same. I wondered how Tom was, and if this would work. We all cried a bit, talked a bit, but mostly kept quiet and waited. After several hours Dr. Ellenbogen came out to talk with us.

Dr. Ellenbogen was dressed in his operation clothes, a white non-descript robe draped over his pale blue surgical scrubs. He wore a brightly colored hat that fit tight around his head to keep all his hair in. He walked in and started talking. He told us the surgery was going well. Tom had not lost much blood and his vital signs were strong. Then he showed us a picture of inside of Tom's head and explained what he had removed.

Surprisingly, the tumor had taken over all of the right side of Tom's cerebellum, the part of the brain that should control Tom's movement, mostly fine motor skills, on the right side of his body. He showed us the pictures of the tumor and how big it was, but I really could not tell what I was looking at. But I was there because of Dr. Ellenbogen and he had my trust. With that trust he had removed the entire cerebellum on the right side of Tom's brain.

Dr. Ellenbogen informed us that great trauma had already been done to the area he had to remove, and that the left side of Tom's cerebellum must already be compensating for the damaged right. He thought Tom might lose some movement control but overall he would be about the same as before the surgery. The part of the tumor that concerned him the most was the part that had attached itself to the brain stem. He had gotten as much as he could and now we would have to trust the radiation team.

The surgery was finished and Tom had done well. Mom, dad, Beth and I were allowed into the recovery room to see him as he woke up. Tom is very high strung and our presence was meant to calm him.

Hormones and Drugs

Anesthesia does weird things to your mind as you wake up. When I had back surgery I was told that I screamed obscenities as I was coming out of the fog, but I never remembered it. Tom's reaction, as a boy that was getting ready to be 15, was what we should have expected but had no idea was coming.

"Where's the nurse!" Tom yelled in a loud voice. "I know she is here, can you see my dick swinging? Where is the nurse, she is so hot. Nurse!"

Beth did not know what to say and mom did this odd combination of flushing and turning red all at the same time. It only took them a minute to decide to leave until Tom was more lucid. I know Tom was hurting, I knew that he did not know what he was saying and I knew that it was not a good time but I just could not help myself, and I laughed. For a solid minute I laughed a deep, belly laugh. Dad just chuckled a moment and said "Randy" in what was meant to be a sobering voice.

Tom was in the hospital for ten days this time as they monitored his progress, checked for infection, and he learned how to use his legs again. He was given pain medications through his IV, others in pill form, and he also had a drip, where he could push a button when he was in pain and Dilaudid would be pushed through his veins by a machine that carefully measured and administered each dose. Tom recovered quickly as he had in the past, but he was only part way though this time. Soon he would start the horror of radiation.

Fires, Friends and the Search for Peace

Waiting is tough; all you can do is hope. We could not do much and Beth and I searched for moments of peace. We searched for ways to forget, to laugh, to find the very elusive peace. I don't remember which of us came up with the idea but I think we were together when we bought the large copper, outdoor fire pit. We set it up in the back yard and began lighting the fires of peace.

The first time we lit the fire pit we invited the neighbors and they came. We provided the fire, music and drinks. It did not take long for the invitations to become unnecessary, I lit the fire and they would come.

Larry and Rema lived directly behind us. Larry was a police officer and Rema a dispatcher. I thought Larry was joking when he suggested we cut a hole in the fence so we could let the dogs play and we could visit easier, at least I thought he was joking until I heard the saw.

Scott and Melissa lived to the south side of us. Scott worked for Boeing and Melissa worked for the local school and coached javelin throwing when she was not attending to their five kids. These made up the neighbors that were at most every fire. We would also have several others from time to time, the gate and doors were always open.

Radioactive

After Tom had healed from the surgery for some time he was ready to begin radiation. The first step was to talk with the doctors about what to expect and to have his head measured and molded. A tight fitting mask was made from a rigid plastic that could be fastened to the radiation table in the same spot. Once the mask was made Tom was placed on the table and x-rays were taken of the exact position that Tom would be in. Then a plan was developed.

The chief radiologist had to create a plan for the exact placement, strength and duration of each beam of radiation. He would then submit the plan to the physicist who would validate whether the radiologist's plan could actually be completed with the equipment. If changes needed to be made, the physicist would suggest the solution that would go back to the radiologist, and the processes would start again. It took almost two months for the actual radiation treatment to begin.

Tom received radiation three times a week. The first few trips were pretty easy and he did not seem to suffer too many effects, but after a couple of weeks the nausea set in, and it was brutal. Every time he would throw up it would cause waves of intense pain in his already aching head. He was already thin and weak and now he could not keep food down. Most of the anti-nausea medications had little effect and Tom's appetite was limited. He began to lose more weight and he lost it quickly. He was getting dangerously thin.

Tom was now over six foot tall and he weighed 115 pounds. The doctors began talking about inserting a feeding tube directly into his stomach or through his nasal passage and into his stomach. He could not lose any more weight. In an attempt to increase Tom's weight and avoid such drastic measures, I created the Shake. The Shake was made out of six ounces of heavy cream, Carnation Instant Breakfast, and Dove ice cream. I used Dove ice-cream because it had natural, high calorie, ingredients. I used the Carnation Instant Breakfast because it contains vital vitamins and I used the heavy cream for even more calories. Each twelve ounce Shake contained more than 1500 calories and Tom drank at least three a day, usually four. During radiation therapy Tom actually gained fifteen pounds.

Tom lost his hair on the right side of his skull where the radiation was beamed. It quickly became very shaggy and he was ready to have all his hair cut so it would at least look even. We had a hair cutting night at our house. Beth was gentle as she used clippers to cut Tom's hair. Tom was not quite as gentle as he cut off mine. Fortunately, Beth was there to get the spots that Tom missed. After several weeks the radiation stopped but the effects increased. Over the next four months Tom would spend almost all his time inside his room with all the light blocked out. We spent hours at the doctors, the neurologist, and the pain center to find a solution. After more than three years we had tried dozens of different drugs, injections, patches and other methods of administration. Still, Tom was hurting and fighting nausea.

Medical Marijuana Friends

We were visiting with the neurologist at Children's and we had exhausted almost every option. Tom was taking heavy doses of opiates and I was concerned about the addictive properties and so was the neurologist. He tried to explain that Tom might be reliant on the opiates, but it would not be addiction because he had a real need, but even he seemed to have trouble with that line of reasoning. Finally, when we were alone he said "Mr. Dahl, I can't legally suggest this but you might try THC." I was confused and he could tell. He went on and said some people have found that marijuana has been effective in fighting pain and nausea, though it is not approved by the FDA and he could not prescribe it.

I knew I had friends that used it but I did not like the idea of marijuana. To me medical marijuana was just a ruse used by stoners that just wanted to get high But this was my son and I was ready to try anything.

I called Rich. He was the only person I knew that I could reach out to and ask about pot. I had seen him use it so he had to know where I could get some. I expected to have to eat some preverbal crow after all the crap I gave him on our camping trip, and since, but I felt like I had no choice.

Rich and his friends answered the call. I was not given any grief or asked to eat any crow. I was just given what I needed to try and help Tom, with nothing asked for in return. Rich will tell you that is what he did because it is the only right thing to do.

I had never smoked pot. I had heard you can put it into brownies and eat it and so that is what I did. I made a batch of extra chocolate brownies and mixed about one quarter ounce of the pot directly into the brownies and cooked them. I had not real idea of what I was doing but I was going to give it a try.

The next day we made a trip to Oregon to visit family and I gave Tom a large brownie and told him to eat it. He complained of the gritty taste and the vitamin or protein powder, or whatever I was using this time the make him gain weight, but he ate it. About an hour into the time Tom fell asleep in the car, and he slept at my parents' house for the rest of the night.

Tom woke up the next morning in good spirits and told me "Dad, I don't have a headache". That was the first time he had not had a headache in more than four months!

I did not need to give Tom brownies each time he had a headache or went through surgery. Once the cycle of the headache was broken we would be able to keep it in check with other medications. I did utilize the brownies from time to time, but he never knew what was in them until after he was eighteen.

We spent a great deal more time with doctors in the pain clinic trying to find solutions to the headaches. Over time we would try a virtual pharmacy of drugs, including antidepressants, muscle relaxers, and drugs that are meant to slow the pain receptors. The most common solution seemed to be OxyContin and Vicodin. I was concerned about the side effects, including the exacerbation of his nausea, but the overriding issue was controlling his pain enough for him to function.

Chapter 17 - The American Cancer Society

It was Thanksgiving Day of 2005 and I was unemployed. Arvado had gone through dramatic changes, including three presidents of our division, and I finally got caught in the layoffs. Tom was sitting back, reading the newspaper, looking for an after school job, when he said "Dad, why don't you just work for the American Cancer Society?" He was looking at an advertisement for a CRM, Community Relationship Manager, and I thought, I don't know, why not?

The next Monday I called David Allen, the only person that I knew that worked at ACS. I told him about the ad Tom found and that it sounded interesting to work at ACS, and I asked him what he thought about it. He started laughing on the phone, and as I remember it, he laughed for several minutes before he could ask, really, are you serious? I told him I was and he said the CRM position would not interest me but he knew what might and he would set me up.

A few days later I met with Linda, the Region VP for Region 8 of ACS, and the Seattle and Tacoma area. Linda and I went to lunch and her overriding question was "really, are you sure you want to do this?" She also added that they would not pay me as much as I had been making, only about half. The position was VP of Operations and I wanted it. I went through two more interviews and the response was similar, was I sure I wanted this job. It really seemed like they were warning me and trying to talk me out of it. It was the most bizarre process I had been through.

I consulted my friend Rich as I was going through this process and he gave me some thoughts to consider. "Randy, this place is really messed up and underperforming. You can really make it grow but they are not like us. It won't be long before you drive them crazy and they drive you nuts. This will not be long term for you." Charles, the Chief of Staff at the time, told me he looked at my resume and told them to hire me. I was what they needed, and he did not need to meet me. And so I joined the American Cancer Society.

Not long after I joined, Linda left ACS and I was promoted to Region VP. I understood that this was a service organization, that we needed to be personable, and Region 8 was cold impersonal name, so our team started referring to our region as the Puget Sound Region. It was interesting, it caused a great deal of flack, but soon every region had a name instead of a number.

I needed an Executive Director for the northern part of the region and I asked Christi Beckley, an employee that was recognized as a leader, to take the promotion. She declined. I interviewed a few more people, then asked Christi again and she declined again. I did one more round of interviews and asked Christi if she would please take the position and she finally did.

Tom, the Executive Director in Tacoma changed jobs to working with corporations and major accounts. David Stickland was on the team in Tacoma and I had gotten to know him and his passion. He had survived childhood cancer and the bones in his right leg had been replaced with titanium. There was not much that would stop, or even slow down David, so I asked him to work with me as the ED in Tacoma.

Rachel Kirk was a Quality of Life Manager and had been with ACS for seven years. She has a grand and open heart and a great understanding of the things--many of them little things--that cancer survivors desperately need. As quickly as I could I promoted Rachel to the Executive Director of Quality of Life, moving the service mission of the ACS forward.

Our team was strong and focused, and we grew as a team. We had a singular desire to support those fighting against the cancer demon, providing needed support, helping volunteers organize, and raising money to fund research. In four years, we grew services alone by providing assistance to over 8,000 survivors a year in our Puget Sound Region, up from 798. And on my white board, and in my home, there was always the quote visible, "Randy, can you work faster please?"

Shortly after I joined the ACS I met Terry Wilcox. I was attending a volunteer meeting for Relay For Life in Auburn and Terry was there. When I introduced myself Terry engaged me with passion and concern. She quickly unloaded a vast array of needs of the volunteers that she felt were not being met by the ACS staff and management and her views of how we could do so much more. I was a little shocked, taken aback, and I admired the passion that she displayed. I wondered, were all the volunteers like this? If so, this would be difficult to manage, but if we could support that potential it would be nothing less than amazing.

Go Faster and Not Fast Enough

Terry's husband Clark was a police sergeant with the Kent Police Department. He oversaw the motorcycle officers and he rode a Honda Goldwing on his personal time. Terry rode her own Kawasaki cruiser, and she was aware that I rode a Honda Aero, another cruiser. Terry gave me a call and invited me on a ride in late September that she was putting together at the request of a cancer Survivor. It was on this ride that I met Audrey.
Audrey was a slight woman with short curly grey hair. She was in her early sixties and had never smoked and had lived a healthy lifestyle. Nevertheless, she had developed lung cancer. While talking with her friends she had mentioned that she had never ridden on a motorcycle and would like to have a ride on a Goldwing someday. That message made its way to Terry and on this day in September Terry organized a ride with Clark on his Goldwing, Audrey his passenger, and 20 motorcycles following behind.
Three friends came to the party that day with Audrey and joined the ride. The first two of her friends rode with two of Clark's officers on big Harley Davidson motorcycles, following directly behind Clark and riding side by side. The third friend of Audrey's rode with me, a woman in her fifties with a great smile, who had never been on a motorcycle in her life.

I followed as Clark led the group through slow turning roads, winding their way through trees, along rivers, and past green fields filled with flowers and livestock. The trip was beautiful and we stopped after an hour of riding at a small town that I had not visited before. As we were getting ready to start our way back, Audrey asked Clark if he could ride faster, and off they went.

Clark and his officers took off with their passengers and I tried to follow with mine. They were much better, and more experienced riders than I am and they had much more powerful bikes. My passenger was not a natural on a motorcycle and had difficulty leaning into the turns with the bike but gave in to the temptation to lean out the other way, making the ride more difficult. I tried my best to keep up with Clark and I focused completely on that for several miles. We passed some fields, crossed some roads, and climbed some hills, all in rapid succession. As we made our way out of one curvy, tree lined area and came to a long straight stretch of road I noticed Clark and his officers were nowhere in sight. I looked in my rearview mirror and noticed no one was behind us either, and neither I nor my passenger knew where we were. So we just kept riding.

Eventually we came to large gravel parking area where Clark, Audrey, and the other four people we were following were off their bikes and waiting for us. They had been waiting for several minutes. I pulled over and we got off my bike and started talking to the speed demons and several minutes later the rest of the posse showed up.

We finished the ride back at the Wilcox's home where a BBQ lunch was waiting. It was then that Terry introduced me to Audrey, telling her that I was the Region Vice President for ACS. Audrey gave me a hug and whispered in my ear, "Randy, can you work faster please?"

I could not work fast enough for Audrey and she passed away two months later from lung cancer. That question both inspires me and haunts me every day, and I think about Audrey, Terry, Clark, and the many people that I was fortunate to serve with at ACS.

Picture of Success

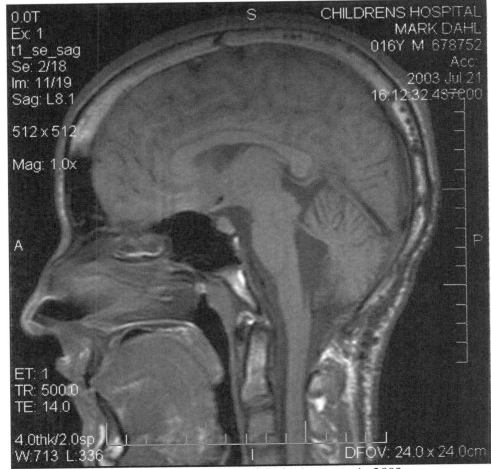

MRI of Tom's head showing the return of the brain tumor in 2003.

I carried the picture up to the podium and stood in front of the crowd of 88 people that had purchased tickets to the Camp Goodtimes Wine Auction. It was a formal event and this was in the middle of the live auction. The money raised through most of the auction went to fund Camp Goodtimes, a week long camp for kids that were cancer Survivors. But this auction item was different, item number 16, a paddle raise to fund scholarships for childhood cancer Survivors.

The framed picture was wrapped in black velvet and tied with a golden lace bow. Beth had helped me take the time to carefully wrap it so that it would not be damaged, and have a covering representative of the value of the art inside.

"I want to thank you for coming here and participating in our event tonight" I began. I could feel the emotions well inside me as I continued. "Tonight I have the opportunity to share with you the most valuable piece of art I have ever owned. It is a piece of modern art that took years to craft. It is unique in that it took many artists, and craftsmen to create it, each of them studying many years to perfect their craft, all of them dedicating their entire life to their piece."

"As I look at this piece it evokes extreme emotions, and hope that it has this effect for you, too. An artist's work has to evoke emotion, and this particular piece has done an exceptional job of capturing the yin and yang of life." As I was talking I was carefully, slowly, untying the gold ribbon, and taking care to unwrap it neatly so I could place it on the podium.

"This picture was created with great care, and using a combination of art, tools, and technology that has not existed at any other time in history. As such, it has captured a view of demons that dwell in the soul--of fear, pain, heartache, and a darkness completely void of hope. But as you search the fine detail and look deeper into the piece you will see triumph over the demons. You will see light, hope, dedication and love. "

Hidden by the podium I removed the fine velvet wrapping, carefully folded it, and placed it beside the gold ribbon that had recently held it together.

"As you continue to study this picture you will realize that it tells an amazing story of the past and present, and it even shows the future. Though it is done in black and white it screams of color and life. Though it took years and vast sums of money to create, it is priceless. This item is not for sale this evening, but I want to share it with you in my desire to help you understand the hope and the life it represents, and your part in creating the picture and all of the things it represents."

I lifted up the framed picture to show the crowd and explained. "These are MRI images of my son, Tom's brain. On the left you can see this large enhanced area that shows white, and these large, long, dark places that seem to block out what should be his brain. The white area is a tumor, doing its best to trap fluids in his head, a demon guarding the path to freedom and life. The large, long, dark places are the fluid, expanding, crushing the life from his mind and body. The demons fighting for control, causing loss of hope and life."

"On the right, you can see an MRI scan of Tom's brain four years later. This was taken six months ago. Now there is a dark hole where the demon tumor was and the ventricles are back to normal size, you can see how the compressed brain matter has returned to a normal size and shape. You can see the work of the craftsmen, the doctors and nurses that dedicated their life to put on the armor and battle such demons. You will appreciate the work of the scientists that sacrifice so much to focus on minute details and create the weapons for the knights to use in battle. And you can read the future in the notations on the bottom of the picture; the tumor is showing no signs of enhancement."

"Ladies and gentlemen, a picture paints a thousand words and it is my pleasure to introduce you to the hero in this picture and story, my son, Tom Dahl".

Everyone stood and applauded as Tom made his way to the podium, most with tears in their eyes. Tom stood in front of the group and told them of the challenges of high school while fighting cancer. How he had missed essentially two years of being with his class, but through the help of Beth, tutors, and a great many teachers he was able to graduate, and only six months behind the rest of his class. He told them he knew the financial burden that his care had placed on his family and yet he knew he needed a college education, perhaps more than others, to compensate for the disabilities that he would be left with. He told him of his dream, to work with special needs kids in elementary schools and day cares. When Tom finished the crowd once again rose to their feet and applauded. As he walked back to the table where we were seated several people gave him hugs and shook his hand. As he got close to our table Beth threw her arms around him, tears streaming down her face, and told him how proud of him she was.

The auctioneer returned the podium, commented on Tom's story, and asked people to raise their paddles to give to fund scholarships for kids that had battled cancer and wanted to attend college. In a matter of moments $30,000 was raised.

Tom never received a scholarship, but he still works to use his gifts to help others with special needs get an education.

Chapter 18 - MS

It was May, and Karee was excited. A talented and energetic staff member, she had heard about the Charity Runner program, and was busy finding volunteers to run marathons and raise money for the American Cancer Society. She already had 4 events, the most of any of my team members, but she wanted to start one in Seattle. We already had less than the year typically recommended for set-up, including recruiting teams, training, and raising money, but Karee was excited and I was not going to stand in her way. Besides, I had this weird thing going on with my mouth and jaw and arguing was not fun.

Karee worked hard and recruited teams to run and raise money. She had found a corporate sponsor and a fitness trainer that would teach our runners the art of Chi Running. ChiRunning is a form of running using the principles of tai chi to focus on alignment, relaxation and proper form when running and walking with an emphasize posture, core strength, relaxed legs, and "mindfulness". I agreed that if she managed the program, I would run the marathon and do a personal fund raising effort for the event in November. This was crazy--who thought up the notion that running 26.2 miles was a good idea, and who in Seattle thought it would be a good idea to do it on Thanksgiving weekend? Oh well, I had run marathons before and I could do it again. I had completed a marathon the year after Tom's first surgery. I had used running to find peace and fight stress, and had thought that my last marathon had been just that, my last marathon. But I would do one more to support Karee, Survivors and ACS.

At first I was not sure if it was the running or what, but I was getting odd cramps, spasms really, down my right side. They hurt, but they did not last long, only about twenty seconds, and it only happened every couple of days. The running and stress was messing up my taste buds too. Nothing tasted good, actually most things tasted nasty, and I felt like I had a thick layer of slime on my tongue.

The spasms grew in frequency and pain. They still only lasted about twenty seconds, but they were occurring about every hour, even while I was sleeping. I was not getting sleep and I was getting cranky. Beth was concerned and suggested I see a doctor, but I had a great deal to do and I really did not have time.

I was losing some focus at work. I had to slow down with my speech and my thoughts, they just weren't coming as fast as they needed to. It seemed to take me more time to process what people were saying and I had to work to get the words out to respond. It was irritating and scary. I knew that the nervous system works from the brain down and the pain extended all the way down my right side, starting at my jaw. My thoughts were slowing and my responses were also delayed. I had seen the challenges Tom had with his right side and I began to fear that I was developing a tumor as well.

I hid the challenges and put it off as long as I could. By now, the spasms were happening at least every twenty minutes and the pain was excruciating. I could not sit in a meeting without showing obvious pain and several members of my team were nagging me to see a doctor.

I had delayed as long as I could. The pain was getting too great and no medications I had were doing anything. It was late June when I finally made an appointment to see Jack, our family doc.

Jack examined me, asked me questions, and did a series of tests to show my balance abilities. I would not have passed a roadside sobriety test, though I had stopped almost all drinking. After a while, Jack came to the same conclusion that I had, something was wrong with my nervous system and a tumor was likely. He scheduled me for an MRI the next day.

Later that day I had a meeting with Stephanie, my boss at the American Cancer Society. As with everyone else, she could see something significant was wrong. I shared what my doctor had said and she turned stern and told me, "Randy, you have connections, you have ability to pull strings with the best doctors. Pull them, use what you have, and get this taken care of now!"

The pain and thoughts of tumors and cancer weighed heavily on my mind. At about 9:30 that night, I sent an email message to Dr. Marc Stewart, the Medical Director for Seattle Cancer Care Alliance and a member of the Leadership Council that guided me at ACS. I was shocked when just a few minutes later, I received a reply, and just a few minutes after that, we were talking on the phone.

I explained to Dr. Stewart what had been happening. He listened, asked a few questions and suggested that I send a note to Dr. Ellenbogen and ask his opinion. After we hung up, I sent a similar message to Dr. Ellenbogen, and again, I was shocked when the phone rang just a few minutes later.

Dr. Ellenbogen listened to me. Then he told me when I had my MRI the next morning, to ask for a copy of it on a CD, take the CD to his office at Harborview, and give it to his assistant who would download the images on the system where he could look at them. He was currently in Chicago, returning on Saturday. It took me a minute to realize he was calling me at midnight where he was.

It was Friday, and the MRI went smoothly. I received a copy, made an appointment with Jack for a follow up on Monday afternoon, and then left for Harborview. It was about noon when I met Dr. Ellenbogen's assistant and gave her the CD.

Friday evening, Dr. Ellenbogen called me and told me that he had looked at my files but the pictures were kind of blurry. He was flying home on Saturday and he would look at them from there, where he had a larger monitor.

On Saturday, he called me and said that the images were still fuzzy, that he would have to go in and pull the images from the disk directly. He would call me Monday morning. When he hung up I was getting more concerned. There was something there; that was obvious. What I was waiting for was how bad it was, and that sucked.

Dr. Ellenbogen did not wait for Monday. It was Sunday morning when he called. "Randy, I can tell you that you don't have a tumor or brain cancer, but you do need to see a neurologist. I am a neurosurgeon, so I can't tell you that you have multiple sclerosis, but you do. I am sorry to have to tell you this, but you need to see a neurologist as soon as you can.

I have MS. I have no idea what that means but a neurosurgeon, the neurosurgeon that has operated on my son's brain, that fights cancer, is telling me he is sorry. I had no idea what was happening but I was feeling sick inside.

My first thought was to turn to Wikipedia:

"MS affects the ability of nerve cells in the brain and spinal cord to communicate with each other effectively. Nerve cells communicate by sending electrical fibers called axons, which are contained within an insulating substance called myelin. In MS, the body's own immune system attacks and damages the myelin. When myelin is lost, the axons can no longer effectively conduct signals. The name multiple sclerosis refers to scars (sclerae-—better known as plaques or lesions) particularly in the white matter of the brain and spinal cord, which is mainly composed of myelin. Although much is known about the mechanisms involved in the disease process, the cause remains unknown. Theories include genetics or infections. Different environmental risk factors have also been found."

"Almost any neurological symptom can appear with the disease, and the disease often progresses to physical and cognitive disability. Psychiatric symptoms may also occur. MS takes several forms, with new symptoms occurring either in discrete attacks (relapsing forms) or accumulating over time (progressive forms). Between attacks, symptoms may go away completely, but permanent neurological deficits often occur, especially as the disease advances."

"There is no known cure for multiple sclerosis. Treatments attempt to return function after an attack, prevent new attacks, and prevent disability. MS medications can have adverse effects or be poorly tolerated, and many people pursue alternative treatments, despite the lack of supporting scientific study. The prognosis is difficult to predict; it depends on the subtype of the disease, the individual's disease characteristics, the initial symptoms and the degree of disability the person experiences as time advances. Life expectancy of people with MS is 5 to 10 years lower than that of the unaffected population."

The more I read the more questions I had. The next day I saw Jack, who reviewed my MRI report and told me he was sorry, I had MS. He would set me up with a neurologist as soon as possible but it would likely be four to six weeks. He explained that that was rushing it.

The spasms continued and my mind hurt. I began to read stories about people with MS, that it can cause you to lose control of your legs, your mind, your bladder and can result in death. Tom was just healing, I had work to do, was I going to die in constant pain? Even as I had these thoughts the pain spread through my side. It took my breath, it was a message loud and clear "YOU ARE FUCKED."

The next day was a Tuesday and it started with my Leadership Council meeting. I can't tell you what happened during the meeting, but after the meeting I was cornered. Dr. Stewart from SCCA and Dr. Einstein and Dr. Labrolia from Swedish Hospital asked me what was going on. I told them my story, that I had MS, and they all sunk a little bit and said "Randy, I am so sorry". What was going on? How bad was this MS crap? Some of the best cancer docs in the nation are telling me that they are sorry to hear I am so sick. Can this be worse than cancer? Damn.

The Leadership Council meeting lasted until 9:00. At 10:00 I received a call from Dr. Labrolia. He and Dr. Einstein had talked to the Neurosciences clinic at Swedish and I had an appointment with Dr. Larry Murphy at 2:00 that day. "Don't be late".

It was July 2 when I met Dr. Murphy. He assured me that there are many treatments for MS and that I would get all the care I needed. He provided me with phone numbers and his e-mail address and let me know that he would respond within a day to e-mail; he almost always responds within hours. He set me up with the start of steroid infusions the next day, and that thankfully, quickly subdued my symptoms. I talked to him about my commitment to run the Seattle Marathon in November and he cautioned me to remember that the concrete is harder than my knees and elbows.

I still did not know what was really going on. I was suffering from a combination of depression, fear, pain, and stress. The odd thing is that when your mind is not working right, it takes time to be able to recognize it. It is not like a broken limb where you can see the cast, and as the pain faded from my side it took time to realize what the combination of the disease and stressors had done to my thoughts and resulting actions. And as tough as it was for me, it was likely more difficult for those around me.

The challenges of suffering from chronic diseases, and not understanding them, often leads to stressors in relationships. One of the challenges with MS is the way it affects decision making. This can be caused by the disease itself, or depression and stress caused by the disease. Many times this causes negative actions and problems within families, and it is not uncommon that this may lead to divorce. As I think back today, I am convinced that the effects of MS played a significant role in my separation and eventual divorce from Beth.

Be Thankful

Cynthia worked with me at American Cancer Society, though she served at the division level, managing Quality of Life Programs. She worked to assure that each region maintained a focus on the mission goals and implemented best practices, keeping an eye on key indicators and outcomes. When Cynthia learned that I was battling MS she introduced me to a friend of hers, Dr. Craig Smith. Dr. Smith had spent a great deal of his career focusing on leading edge research into MS, the cause and treatments. A tall, fit man in his sixties, he had been on the National Championship Rowing team at the University of Washington with Dr. Paul Ramsey, now the CEO of the University of Washington Medical Center. The men still row and compete today.

I first met Dr. Smith at a Starbucks coffee shop in Madison Park, an upscale Seattle neighborhood on the west shore of Lake Washington. Dr. Smith was concerned, open, and we discussed the initial options I had for managing my disease. We talked about treatment and he agreed with the recommendations of Dr. Murphy and my personal choices. Then we talked about my interactions with others.

Dr. Smith suggested that there were two effective ways managing my communication and relationships with others. The first would be to not let anyone know except family and my medical care staff. The second would be to embrace it and be extremely open with it. He did not recommend one choice over the other, just that I make a choice. By the end of our conversation my choice was clear to me, I am open, have led an open life, and this would be no different. It would take some time before I learned the challenges that come with this decision.

A few weeks later, Dr. Smith invited Beth and me up to his home on Whidbey Island for dinner. His wife had been an ICU nurse at Children's Hospital in Seattle when Tom was a recovering from some of his surgeries.

The home is set along a beautiful, walkable section of the Puget Sound. The tide was rising as we ate wild Chinook salmon they had bought from a local market and cooked outside on a grill. After dinner and wine we took a walk along the water where Dr. Smith shared his thoughts with me and gave me shocking, and at the time I thought patronizing, advice. "Randy, you need to learn not only to embrace the fact that you have MS, you need to be thankful for it."

I understood the concept. There were experiences and people I would not have had if I had not contracted this disease. I expected the comment to be followed with a religious message that did not come. His advice was practical, but I thought it was also crazy. I already had enough issues to deal with and concerns with Tom. The stress in life was already boiling over and this crap hurt. Why would I be thankful for something that would likely cripple me and cause me a whole host of other challenges?

It took me four years to realize that gift I was given with MS. Through my dealing with MS, the challenges, the reactions of others, and the days of lethargy, depression and the uncertainty of what is going to happen next, I have learned to understand my son more and the struggles he has every day in life. I think I have also been better at relating to him, working with him, and helping him heal when needed to find progress and joy in life.

At first I thought he was nuts, but today I know he was right. Dr. Smith gave me extremely valuable gift with his time, and with advice that I continue to reflect on often.

Chapter 19 - Charity Runner

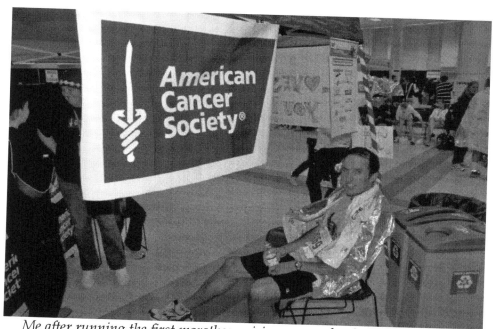

Me after running the first marathon raising money for the American Cancer Society.

The fatigue and depression were challenging. I was still running and trying to decide if I was going to indeed run in the Seattle Marathon. I was pretty sure I could when I was talking to Tom about it and he said "Dad, if I can survive nine brain surgeries and relearn to walk, you can run a marathon with MS." He was right. He did not give up and neither would I.

The Charity Runner program was taking off, but Karee wanted more. She wanted to motivate people, so she got in touch with Mary Swift with the Seattle PI. Mary agreed to write a human interest story about the run and asked who might be interesting. Karee asked if they could write about Tom and I, and I agreed. The following story was run in the Seattle PI on November 25, 2008.

WHEN RUNNERS LINE UP on Fifth Avenue for the Seattle Marathon on Sunday, 45-year-old Randy Dahl plans to be among them -- running for the American Cancer Society.

The cause is personal.

And never mind that if he didn't cross the starting line, few would blame him for backing out.

It was July 2000. Dahl and his son, Tom, then 12, were in Utah at a family reunion when Tom suffered a seizure. Dahl rushed him to a small hospital, and after a CT scan, doctors told him Tom had a tumor and was dying. He was rushed to a Salt Lake City children's hospital.

"Five minutes after we got there, they were drilling a hole in his head to relieve the pressure," Dahl says, his voice breaking.

A 13-hour surgery followed. Partway through, a doctor came out. The tumor is on Tom's cerebellum, he told Dahl; there's a chance Tom may never talk or walk again.

"At that point everything went black," Dahl says now. "I couldn't see the next minute in time."

Fast-forward to the ICU. Tom is screaming.

"Dad, it hurts!" he says.

Call it bittersweet music to a desperate father's ears.

"You don't want to hear your kid scream," Dahl says. His voice cracks. He struggles for composure. "But if you didn't know if he was going to talk again. ..."

And some time after that would come what Dahl calls "the dance": Dahl's arms supporting Tom, Tom's feet on Dahl's as they execute a slow waltz around the room.

Tom would learn to walk again. And the tumor, considered benign, would show up again.

There would be nine surgeries.

Despite missing large amounts of school, Tom would graduate from high school just six months later than his graduating class.

Now 21, he lives in his own apartment in Fife, a small piece of the tumor still attached to his brain stem.

"His cognitive skills are fine, but he has ataxia and shakes on the right side," his father says.

Add yet another reason for Dahl's commitment to do the marathon: Shortly after Tom got sick, so did Dahl's mother, an Oregon resident. Doctors diagnosed uterine cancer. Surgery and radiation followed.

Dahl took up running to help handle stress and did three marathons -- two in Portland, one in Vancouver.

He's easy to pick out when he does a marathon. He wears a T-shirt Tom decorated for him years ago. On the shirt, two stick figures -- a man and a boy -- cross a finish line together.

Earlier this year, Dahl agreed to run the Seattle Marathon on behalf of the American Cancer Society, not knowing that in July he would be diagnosed with multiple sclerosis.

Any thought Dahl might have entertained about hanging up his running shoes quickly was doused by Tom.

"I beat a brain tumor. You couldn't run 26 miles with MS?" Tom asked, his tone heavy with unmistakable challenge.

Consider it noted.

"I'm going to finish that marathon," Dahl says. "I may crawl across the damn line, but I'm going to finish.

"MS will slow me down a little bit. When I get hot, I lose a little balance. "When everybody else is running 26.2 miles, I'll probably run 29," says Dahl, who became an American Cancer Society volunteer six years ago and is now the organization's vice president for the Western Washington region.

"You think of David and Goliath," he says. "David had a rock. I have a tiny pin.

"I'm going to pick at this giant as long as I can. This thing called cancer went after my family.

"Absolutely, this is personal -- and if it was your kid, it would be personal, too."

Dahl asked me to list this Web site, seattlecharityrunner.org, where readers can make donations to support runners.

"It doesn't have to be me," Dahl says. "It can be for anybody."

I finished the Seattle Marathon, surrounded by a large group of family and friends cheering me on and supporting me at the finish line. Beth, Rich, Terry, Clark and several others came and gave me energy to make it across that final line, and I did not have to crawl. At the end of the event, my friends asked me to join them for lunch and a beer, something that I had done many times in previous marathons. However this time I declined, and without explanation, walked back to my boat. A few other friends were there for a few minutes, and as soon as they left I collapsed on my bed. We raised a hundred thousand dollars. I ran 26 miles. We increased the services for others exponentially and raised dramatically more money for the American Cancer Society and any other time in history, and yet I knew my own son was still struggling. He still hurt, he was "reliant" on addictive and destructive pain medications, and we both struggled.

Rich was right, despite the wild success, the long time chiefs at the ACS did not like the way I worked and pushed and I never learned how to adapt to their culture, so at the end of 2009, we agreed to part ways. My manager continued to look for ways for me to leave, she could have fired me, and I could have quit. In the end we decided that we would separate as an extended part of a previous reduction in force, the ACS term for layoffs. It would only be a few months before the other key members of my team would separate from ACS as well. We had amazing experiences, but it was time to find another avenue to serve, and I would need time for the additional challenges that Tom was going to face and the support he was going to need.

North & South

Learning that I had MS was hard, but not as difficult as learning how to deal with it. Recognizing what it was doing to my mind and how it changed my life was the most challenging and damaging of all.
I had heard about mental illnesses. My sister, Michele, works with the National Alliance on Mental Illness, or NAMI. Her former husband is disabled due to mental illness, and her daughter struggles with it. I knew about depression, fears, and to some extent irrational thoughts. What I did not realize was that it is a side effect--no, a direct effect--of MS, in the most literal sense.
The MS was physically attacking my brain and the way it transmits information, causing short circuiting of sorts. I had felt the spasms that it had caused, and they hurt. That was what had motivated me to see the doctor, but there is a great deal more. One big challenge I was facing was that I did not recognize some very significant effects. How do you know that the basic way you think is affected when the problem is with your own thoughts? Even now that I know, it is sometimes hard to recognize at the time.
For me the greatest challenges were fear, depression and painful lethargy.

The fear and depression are real. First there is the pain; I could not ignore that, at least not all of it. However that is only the beginning. The real fear is about what is coming, or in reality, what may be coming. I don't know the future, but I have seen people with severe MS walking with support canes, in wheel chairs, and fighting to complete basic tasks. Now I know that there are many more people living with MS who I would not even suspect had the disease. My thoughts had slowed. I had to take a bit more time to think things through. Most people, those that do not know me well, assume that I am just being contemplative. What irritates me is that my ability to participate in quick witted banter and high spirited debates has diminished. I was afraid that I was losing my mind, losing *me*, and that I would lose my ability to take care of my family. Beth and Bug could take care of themselves, where would Tom get the support he needs? Would I become a drain on all of their resources?

My life had changed; I was just slow to accept it. The painful lethargy was real and I would need to learn how to deal with it. At the time, I did not know that I could do anything but push through it, so by the time I started heading home from work I would get tired, almost to the point of being unsafe to drive. I was so tired my bones hurt, the kind of pain you feel when you have a really bad case of the flu. And with that came sadness, depression.

Beth and I had been through a lot-- the fear and stress of dealing with a critically sick child, moves, doctors, financial challenges, and family disagreements. Through all of this we had only gotten closer. We did everything together. We searched for ways to fight the pain and stress, to find moments to forget and to lose ourselves in each other. We loved each other deeply, but now we had another challenge that we would not be able conquer. One more major disaster, one more set of challenges, and this time neither of us had enough energy or knowledge to bring us through it together.

It started simply enough. Beth worked for Goodwill in Tacoma, south of where we lived in Milton, about a thirty minute drive. I worked on Queen Anne Hill in Seattle, about an hour drive north of our home, ninety minutes during rush hour. Many nights by the time I got home I hurt, and it was like bending iron to get moving in the morning. I felt stiff, like I had just played football for hours the night before, though the last time I had played football was in high school. So I looked for a place to sleep a few nights a week close to my office. What I found was a boat.

Beth and I had been in Vancouver, British Columbia, and we were looking over the bay at the boats when we decided to get a boat that I could stay on. As we drove home we stopped in Bellingham where we found a 40 foot Sea Ray, and we both loved it. We bought it and it allowed me to spend nights in the north while Beth stayed in the south, and the distance in our relationship would grow with devastating consequence.

I spent many nights alone on the boat, most of the time drinking, staring out at the beauty of the city and trying to numb the pain and the thoughts. Some nights a friend or two would stop by and we would talk, laugh, or go to the restaurant on the corner of the dock for happy hour. I missed Beth, was unreasonably angry with her for not being with me, and at times did not want her with me. I felt that I needed her to hold on, be strong, even as I was withdrawing and pushing away.

We had been through so much together, and now we were separate people living our own lives. After fifteen years of marriage we had become cold, and divorced in just a matter of months.

Chapter 20 - To a New Life of School

His pain had been almost unbearable. Tom's friends had made his place a crash pad. It had become a place to drink, smoke pot, and take pills. The apartment was a mess and it had been broken into more than once by people looking for Tom's pills or other mind altering objects. When Tom tried to clean up, or ask his friends to not do drugs or drink at his place, they became angry, violent and destructive. Many of them did not care if he was hurting and needed quiet. They did not really believe that he was hurting any more than they were.

It was in the middle of July and Tom was living in an apartment in Fife, Washington. He was a young man, 21, and he needed to have his space, grow, take care of himself, and be as much like other young adults as possible. I provided him with assistance with rent and food, but he managed his day to day tasks. He had graduated from Fife High School, worked a couple of part time jobs, but now he was not doing much. He was feeling unproductive, depressed and the people that surrounded him thought of him as a guy with a place to party, and who had pain medications that they could sneak from time to time. He was feeling in a rut and he needed to do something to change that.

I had been encouraging Tom to go to college, possibly in Tacoma at the University of Washington or Evergreen Community College and he had been considering what he wanted to do, but was having trouble deciding and finding motivation. The cycle of depression was difficult to break. With the depression came lack of motivation, and that accentuated the ever present lethargy, which fed the depression even more. All this was in addition to the constant and chronic headaches. To combat the headaches Tom relied on OxyContin, the opiate that has an additional side effect as a depressant. The cycle was brutal.

It was about noon when Tom called. "Dad", he started out, "I know what I want to do." He had a lively tone in his voice and seemed excited. But then I began to doubt when he said, "I want to move to Oregon." My immediate reaction was "why?" Moving to Oregon would be expensive, I would not be able to give him the support I felt he needed, and then there was the medical care, but I let him continue.

"I want to move to Oregon to go to school" he continued. "I want move to Gresham and go to Mt. Hood Community College. Grandma and Grandpa live close by, my cousins Chris and Jake live by the school and are taking classes there, and my cousin Jeremy is going to school there. All our family is nearby and I would like to get out of here and get a new start."

I am sure that there was more discussion at the time, but in my memory it seemed as though that I was at his door, helping him pack before he got off the phone. Tom was going back to school; he was taking steps to move forward in life.

The next week Tom took the train to Portland where his grandparents picked him up and drove him back to their place to stay for a week. During that time, his cousin Abby drove Tom around to look at apartments close to the school. I am not sure how many they looked at, but they decided on a small apartment settled alongside the Gresham Public Golf Course. Tom loves to play golf, had a full set of clubs, and from there he could walk the mile to school, or take the bus.

While he was there Tom went to the school and registered for classes. The next day his cousin drove him to the train station and he returned home. A few days later we began the move.

Glen is my brother-in-law's nephew. Glen is cheerful and odd in nature and had bought a derelict moving van that needed work on the engine, had made the repairs, and used it to travel in, camp, and at times he would pick up jobs from Craig's List . A giving person he was eager to help Tom pack his stuff and move to Gresham to start his new life and his college adventure.

Glen showed up in Seattle with a fourteen foot long painting in the back of his van. Through Craig's List he had found an artist who paid him to deliver the painting to a new, upscale restaurant in downtown Seattle. Glen picked me up; we found the address and delivered the painting. He spent the night with me on the boat and the next morning we were off to Tom's apartment to make the move.

Tom had a kitchen table and chairs, a large flat screen television, a bed, clothes, a few kitchen supplies, his cat and several bags and boxes that were filled with I don't know what, but we fit it all in the van. I followed behind Gen and his van as we made the three hour drive to Tom's new place in Oregon and his new life as a college student. Tom felt good, but I think I was the one who was really excited.

The apartment that Tom had chosen was on the second floor of the apartment building. Located in the back of the complex, he had a nice view of the golf course. My father and his cousin Chris had come by to help us unload the van and carry the large items to the top of the stairs. At the end of the day Tom had a new place and a new beginning on life.

The trips to the hospital for surgeries were tough, disheartening, and difficult to deal with. The memories of the pain were almost as bad. Then came the many trips to the emergency room when the pain got too horrible to bear. And each trip to the emergency room would bring another set of doctors and nurses that had not seen him before. They would look at the large scars on the back of his skull, listen to him describe the pain and do an X-ray or CT scan. When they received the results they would inevitably be almost paralyzed trying to make a decision on how to treat Tom. They would see the images of the large vacant "hole" in his brain, the metallic valve, and the shunt running down his neck. Most of the emergency room doctors had never seen anything like it.

Next would come the results of the blood tests, and listening to Tom. The levels of opiates in his blood would be highly elevated; by the time he got to emergency he would have taken the maximum prescribed dose of pain medications and usually more. The levels they would see would raise concern that his heart would stop. So any actions, additional drugs, would be slow in coming and Tom would become impatient and increasingly angry. The agitation caused by the opiates, and increased by the pain, would make Tom unbearable and even more difficult to treat. As time passed and he got older he became an even worse patient.

When the additional pain medications came, and were injected into his bloodstream, his agitation would gain strength. He would almost fight the relaxing effects of the medications, and his anger would grow. It was understandable that he was angry with life but it was very difficult to have patience with and to work with. When he would finally calm down and the pain would recede, he would inevitably be given a prescription for additional pain medications. After these events I would take Tom to see pain specialists and we would talk about pain levels, modification, and ways to live with it. His pain pills would be evaluated and strengthened. I would question the addictive properties and we would have a discussion about Tom being reliant on pain medications for the rest of his life. What else could they do? He was trying some alternative therapies but they had little effect. I was very concerned about the side effects of the opiates and the issues that came along with addiction, but I was continually corrected that Tom was reliant, not an addict.

At one time there was a suggestion of injection of Botox into Tom's head. Tom was hesitant but went along with the suggestion and the Botox was administered by a doctor in the pain clinic. The idea was that it would block the nerves and muscle responses that caused his horrific headaches. We had no idea how traumatic the procedure would be.

The doctor made twenty six injections into Toms head. Each injection was painful and produced a significant amount of bleeding. Tom wanted to yell and at a few moments could not help but to let out a cry of pain. He was asked if he wanted them to stop but he had come this far and he was going to finish it, he needed to find some relief. The procedure took almost an excruciating hour to complete and Tom's anxiety was high. In the end it had no effect, positive or negative, just the pain of the shots.

Chapter 21 – Betty

"The Universe gives you what you need, when you need it, rather you want it or not." –Betty

Betty is one of the smartest and most educated people I know. She is a lawyer with a PH.D in molecular biology. The daughter of European immigrants, she was raised in difficult circumstances and learned she had to support and earn her education at an early age. She graduated from a state university on the east coast of the United States and then moved to California to earn her PH.D at the prestigious, liberal and progressive University of California, Berkley.

We spent a few hours in the bar that first night throwing back shots of Jack Daniel's Kentucky Bourbon followed with Coke chasers and getting to know each other. She had done her initial research on tobacco and I worked for the American Cancer Society. She had lived a tough life with little family support and I had the idealistic family with parents that are supportive and still living in the country home where I grew up. She had lived in urban areas and interacted with a wide array of people from the homeless and drug addicted to those in the highest levels of academia and I was just learning how to live in the city. She had never had kids and I had two young adult children, one with major health issues. And Betty was unpredictable and fun.

After that first night we walked to our respective homes, which were only two miles apart. After that night we spent most of the next two years together.

By the time Betty met Tom she had done what she does best and researched his medical diagnosis, learning everything she could about him and how to help him heal. Tom and Betty were friends from the moment they met. She understood him, probably better than I did at times. She understood the pain medicines he had been on, had begun to abuse, and what they did to his body, mind and personality. She had been around it, studied it, and experienced it. All I could do was try to understand as an observer, something that is difficult at best, and most times impossible.

Betty was an advocate to get Tom off the opiate-based pain medications well before anyone else recognized the severe damage they were doing, as well as the potential that they had for doing even more. She is an advocate for the use of medical marijuana, and having experience with it, she knew what it could do for him. Having studied it, she knew the adverse effects and concluded that use of marijuana for controlling his headaches was a much better choice than what he was doing. Through her and her friends I learned how this could help Tom.

Betty talked to people that she had known in California who were involved in the cultivation of marijuana. She related Tom's situation to them and they immediately did what they could to help. Betty and I rode my motorcycle to California and her friends provided me with the marijuana that Tom would need to help his pain. Though Tom no longer uses prescription pain medications or medical marijuana, the people that I have gotten to know there still call from time to time to see he is doing and wish him well.

Over time the differences between Betty and I became more than we could deal with as a family so we went our separate ways. However she still calls, loves Tom and me, and does whatever she can when he needs her. That included allowing him to stay with her when he was in his deepest battle with the pain medications, and coming to Oregon to stay with him when he was recovering from his last surgery.

Tom will tell you that Betty has become family.

Chapter 22 - Two Years of Irony

April 3, 2013. Tom struggled a bit as he got out of bed. It was 8:30 and he had gotten used to sleeping in until noon with nothing to do. Today he had a purpose. He did not really feel the motivation, had not felt motivation for anything really, but he knew he needed to get out of this deep rut in life he was in. So he crawled out of bed. Today he was going back to school.

It was a bright and sunny day, not completely unusual but a bit rare for early spring. The sun had been shinning for the past four days and the barometric pressure had been stable, which was good news as it lessened the constant headache. The temperature was around 65, and after a long winter that seemed warm, without being too hot. It really was a great day and as he got ready, he recognized he was looking forward to going back to school.

Tom put on his best jeans. I had just bought them a few days before at Ross. He other jeans were well worn and had large holes in the right leg. He was glad to have nice clothes to wear. It made him think for just a moment and allow a moment of sadness to grab him, but he would not dwell on it today. He put on his jeans, a nice shirt and his boots. He really liked the boots. And he smiled.

I was excited to take Tom to school. It had been a long road getting here. I was so proud of how far he had come and the strength he was showing. He was no longer smoking and he had not had any type of pain pills or drugs since the first of August. He was tough and he was going to make it through school, no doubt, and no doubt the world would be a better place for it.

Tom was finishing his Associates degree at Seattle Central with plans to transfer to Seattle University in the fall. He was going to help special needs kids get the education and support that they need.

Seattle Central is located next to Seattle University and just two miles from the boat where we lived. There is a bus, he could walk, or he could drive, but he chose to ask me to take him and secretly I was happy he did. I dropped Tom off an hour and a half before class.

After dropping Tom off, I turned the car down Pine and headed towards home. I had gone less than one half mile when an unexpected wave of emotions hit. My eyes filled with tears that I could not stop. I almost could not breathe and seeing to drive was nearly impossible. I was damn near fifty and crying like a little girl, and I could not stop. I loved that damn kid and I was so proud of him. The guilt and sadness of all that he had endured came rushing in and the admiration and respect for his resolve, big heart, and love was overwhelming. GO TOM!

Tom walked to find a barber to get his hair cut. It was important to look good at school. After that he made his way to a store for pencils and a note book. He was on time and he was ready. He only had one class today. It was a long class from 1:00 PM to 4:00 PM. He found the room in the main building, next to the room that he would be going to tomorrow, that was nice. He walked up to the door and there was a sign, "CLASS CANCELED TODAY".

Tom looked at the sign and the first though was "Really?" What a pain in the ass. Then he thought for a moment and said out loud to no one, "It figures" and started to make his was home to the boat.

Two Years to Get to Class

It was February, 2011. I was staying with Tom in Oregon because he was not feeling well and losing weight again. It was a Friday and Tom was significantly sick when he got up for his class at Mt. Hood Community College. It was raining, windy, and cold outside, and he was hurting. He was determined to go to class and forced himself up, and I drove him to school where on the door of his class he found a sign that said "Class is canceled for today". Now besides feeling ill, the severe depression also hit even harder and life just seemed to be spiraling beyond all control.

He had been ill since before Christmas and was having trouble eating, sleeping and even moving. I began staying with him in his apartment to help him through this rough time. I was worried and needed to make sure he was eating and had company. Whatever was going on he just could not shake it.

In January he was still sick and getting worse when he told me "Dad, I have a lump on my testicle and I am bleeding when I pee". He was scared. I had known that all the radiation and treatments he had endured exposed him to a risk of secondary cancer but I did not expect this. We went to see his doctor.

We went to see his doctor the next day and he ordered a blood and urine test that came back negative. He told us he had not seen this before and maybe we should watch it for a week and see what happens. I was going crazy.

Tom complained of severe abdominal pain and could not hold food down. At 6'5" he was an alarmingly skinny 135 pounds. We had been to this general practitioner where he underwent blood tests and examinations that did not show anything abnormal. Now we were fearing testicular cancer. I did not know what to do so I reached out to an expert that I did know.

Dr. Stewart was the Medical Director at Seattle Cancer Care Alliance (SCCA) and served as a counselor to me on the Leadership Council at ACS. SCCA is a world class treatment center and associated with the University of Washington and Fred Hutchinson Cancer Research Center. My respect for Dr. Stewart is unmatched and I still think of him of one of our world's heroes. He had given me advice before, so I sent him the following note asking for his advice and help again.

Dr. Stewart,

I am sorry to bother you but I am in some significant need of advice. My son Tom, 23, who has battled the effects of a brain tumor for 10 years has a new issue.

He is currently living in Oregon and on Saturday he discovered a lump on a testicle and blood in his ejaculate. He went to his GP Monday and the doctor took blood for a CBC and a urinalysis which came back normal. He had a sonogram today and a lump 4.5mm to 5mm was discovered. The GP said that she has not dealt with this before but thought is that it is a spermatocele.

Tom has been having significant nausea and lost significant weight. He was down to 135 at 6'5". We just went in for a MRI on his head 3 weeks ago and everything was unchanged.

Tom's groin pain is moving up his abdomen and the pain is growing over the past few days.

Currently his GP is suggesting he wait a week and see what happens. In your opinion is this a wise course of action or should we seek another opinion? Can you please give me some thought on what our course of action should be? If we wait a week can it cause more issues?
I appreciate your help and thoughts.
Thank you,
Randy

Within twenty minutes I received the following response.

"Hi Randy.
I'm sorry to hear about this. Does he have a medical oncologist? If so and he/she is local, I would contact that person first. Next step would be to see an urologist for a definitive exam and interpretation of the ultrasound. If the pain is severe and progressing, he may need to go to the ER. It may very well be a spermatocele, but it's impossible for me to know. Best comfort would be to see a urologist and go from there.
Let me know how I can help.
Best,
Marc"

I immediately searched for urologists associated with Oregon Health Sciences University (OHSU) and started calling for an appointment. It only took a few phone calls and we had an appointment at an office in Portland the next day, but it seemed slow and it was taking forever. I knew that panic was setting in but that neither made it easier to control, nor easier to stay calm around Tom.

Spermatocele, also known as a spermatic cyst, are typically painless, noncancerous, fluid filled cysts that are outpocketing of fluid from the epididymis. It is thought that they are present in up to 30% of men, mostly undetected, and harmless.

The next week we went to have more examinations, x-rays and tests, everything came back negative. The results pointed to a spermatocele, and yet he was just getting sicker.

I kept my girlfriend Isaac, informed of everything that was going on and she responded with love and care. Isaac is surgeon who specializes in treating throat and neck cancers. She was worried about Tom but she also seemed to support everything that the doctors said and I was impatient and questioning. She did her best to keep me calm but I was not in a position to be comforted.

Over the next weeks we would visit more doctors and pain specialists. I questioned how much of this could be a side effect of the massive amount of opiates he was taking for pain. Oxycodone, Norco, Oxytocin, and a varying array of other drugs. He was taking medicines to reduce nausea that were not working, and each medicine seemed to have a side effect of increasing his headaches. Tom was in a spiral.

It was early February and I ventured a trip back to Seattle to see Isaac and check on my boat. Isaac was at the hospital working so I went to the gym, Anytime Fitness in Freemont, to run on the treadmill and reduce some stress.

The men's changing room at the gym was open with a few long benches and grey metal lockers attached to the walls. I brought a gym bag with my shorts and began changing into my running clothes. Part way down the bench was a gentleman that had finished his workout and was putting on a suit. I said something about how it must feel good to be done and he said it was, but now he needed to go back to work. I asked him what he did and he said he was a doctor. I asked what kind of doctor and he said he was a pain specialist at UW, Dr. David Tauben.

I searched for information about Dr. Tauben and found the following information on the University of Washington web site.

"Dr. Tauben is a UW clinical associate professor and director of medical student education in pain medicine in a joint appointment with the Department of Anesthesia and Pain Medicine and Department of Medicine. He provides specialty consultation and care at the Center for Pain Relief."

"He combines specialty skills and experience as both a primary care internal medicine doctor and a pain specialist to diagnose and treat complex and continuing painful conditions. He has particular expertise in the formulation of medication management plans for pain persisting more than three months. He is developing new programs for improved education and training necessary for long-term pain management in the outpatient primary care office setting."

We talked about Tom and his pain and he told me that he would see him but there was a six to eight week wait for an appointment. However, if Dr. Ellenbogen provided a reference he could get him in sooner. I thanked him for his thoughts and went to run on the treadmill.

I had been running for just over a mile when Dr. Tauben came out fully dressed in his suit and ready to return to work. He walked up to me and handed me his card and said "Randy, there is a reason we met here today. If you can get Tom to my office Thursday I will find a way to get him in." I finished my run and was off to get Tom. Tom was hurting but we made the trip up to the UW Pain Center and he visited with Dr. Tauben. They spent almost an hour together and Dr. Tauben took the copies of Tom's medical records that we had kept. He said he would review them and get back to us as soon as possible. We headed back to Oregon because Tom had a class on Friday and he was determined to attend his classes and finish school.

It was raining, windy, and cold outside, and he was hurting. He was determined to go to class and forced himself up, and I drove him to school where on the door of his class he found a sign that said "Class is canceled for today". Now besides feeling ill, the severe depression also hit even harder and life just seemed to be spiraling beyond all control, and it was.

Chapter 23 - 28 Days of ICU

It was a cold and wet Saturday morning when Dr. Tauben called Tom. He had been reviewing Tom's records and his visit, and felt that Tom should undergo a MRI of his head and spine. He explained to Tom that there were some things, though he did not elaborate on what, that can affect the nerves in the spine that can cause a great deal of pain. He explained that in his observation of the pain Tom was enduring that he felt the MRI should take place soon, he would schedule it at Oregon Health Sciences University Hospital in Portland for that evening. Tom was in trouble.

The drive from Tom's apartment to OHSU took about 30 minutes. It was cold, dark, and wet, and Tom was suffering both from pain and severe anxiety. He was smoking some marijuana to both ease the pain and reduce the stress and it did give a little relief, but he was still agitated.

OHSU is a large complex that sets on the side of the West Hills in Portland. At night large parts of the facility are closed and locked so we entered through the emergency room doors. Once inside we asked for directions and wandered through the maze of halls and elevators that took us to the basement where the Radiology department housed the MRI machines. Once there, the technician gave Tom the questionnaire to complete asking about metal, surgeries, pace makers and anything else that might be disrupted by the strong magnetic pull. He filled in the information and noted the programmable shunt in his head and the need to have it reset after the procedure. The technician contacted the neurosurgeon on call to come reset the device when she was done and then escorted Tom back to the machine. She explained that the processes would take about ninety minutes.

Tom had endured more than two dozen MRI scans in the past and was aware of the need to be still while the machine scanned him. The hard surface that he laid on would be uncomfortable to his extremely thin and bony body, while the loud knocking noises of the machine would make his headache even worse than it currently was. He wondered if it could get worse, it was already extremely painful, making him feel like he wanted to give up and just have it all ended, even if he had to die.

He tried, he tried with all his mental and physical ability, but he could not stay still in the MRI. Just staying still hurt, his body ached, and his head was feeling like it wanted to explode. He had no energy left and yet every bone, muscle and cell felt like it was on fire. He wanted to throw up but he did not even have the energy to do that. And so after twenty minutes of trying the technician pulled Tom out of the machine and told us that we would have to reschedule with his doctor and find another option, possibly sedation.

A few minutes after he was pulled from the machine the neurosurgeon, a resident, came into the room to adjust the valve on his shunt. They use a large circular magnet that is placed over the shunt and it provides a reading with an arrow that resembles the workings of a compass. It looks very low tech at first glance. He placed the apparatus over the shunt and made the adjustment and then examined Tom for a minute. After looking at Tom and listening to how he was feeling, he instructed us to go to the emergency room and check in, Tom needed to be watched and there they could address his immediate pain.

Tom was having trouble walking so I found a wheel chair and we made our way up to the emergency room that was filled with 30 or 40 people waiting to be treated. We waited there for 10 minutes until they took us back into a room where he was checked out by a nurse. His blood pressure was a bit high, but his temperature was normal. She asked us a few more questions and left, explaining that the doctor would be in shortly. A few minutes later the doctor arrived.

The doctor examined Tom, listened to his history and asked why he was there. He noticed that Tom seemed to be sweating and took his temperature again, it was spiking and had elevated to 102. He ordered some blood tests and called the neurosurgeon that had reset Tom's shunt valve.

It was about an hour but it seemed like days as Tom began sweating more and complaining of unbearable pain. The tests came back and his white blood cell count was elevated--Tom had an infection. The neurosurgeon came into the room and inserted a small needle into the shunt, at the base of his neck and further down his body to withdraw fluid for testing. The shunt was filled with brain fluid that was draining into Tom's abdomen, working as it was supposed to. The fluid was sent out for testing and again we waited while Tom was started on an IV and given pain and anti-anxiety medications.

The results of the tests came back and we learned that the infection had worked its way into the shunt and was making its way to his brain. Tom was in immediate danger. The neurosurgeon took Tom into a surgical room and gave him local anesthetic as he made small incisions and began to remove the shunt from the lower part of his body. They would try and stop the infection and save the valve that was implanted in his head and brain. It would prove to be a very difficult and painful process; the shunt had been part of Tom for ten years and his body had encapsulated it in calcium, almost making it like cartilage in his body. As soon as that process was done Tom was admitted into ICU where he would continue to fight for his life.

Chapter 24 - Hey Doc

Isaac and I first met in the atrium of the Arnold building of the Fred Hutchinson Cancer Research Center. There is a free standing coffee shop where we ordered the mandatory Seattle latte and sat in the padded chairs to talk. Isaac is a young doctor who had just moved from Alabama and taken her first position as an otolaryngologist, an ear, nose and throat doctor. She specialized in treating cancer at the VA hospitals in Seattle and Tacoma. Being 14 years younger than me and standing 5'10" with short curly, brown hair, and an oversized smile, it seemed odd that she was such an accomplished woman, and in a profession that I regarded with reverence. I was also a bit surprised that she was talking to me and interested in what I had to say.

Isaac was single and the owner of three dogs. I found it very entertaining that one was named Underdog. All the doctors at the Hutch, VA, SCCA, Children's Hospital and Harborview and the University of Washington Medical Center are staffed by the University and are UW employees. This also made Isaac an associate professor. I had a small office and was consulting at the Hutch and through my work with the American Cancer Society I had gotten to know a significantly large group of people in the academic world. She seemed interested and we agreed to have lunch and talk more about Seattle and all it has to offer. I was surprised she agreed to have lunch with me but I was willing to spend as much time as she wanted. She was cute, young and single and I enjoyed talking with her.

It was the end of summer and a great day, so we had lunch at a seafood restaurant just across the road from the Hutch looking out over Lake Union. We dined and talked for over two hours and I really enjoyed it. To this day I don't know why I asked, I was sure she would decline, but there was a party at my friend Richard's house in Issaquah, about 30 minutes away the next night and I asked if she wanted to go. She accepted and we started seeing each other almost every day, even though it would take a month for me to learn how to pronounce otolaryngologist.

Isaac moved to Seattle without knowing anyone, 3,000 miles away from her family in Georgia and Florida. I took her to the Seattle Sounders soccer games, where my friend and I had season tickets in the crazy section of the stands where you sing, chant, and never sit. She loved it. She also enjoyed my boat and exploring the lakes and Puget Sound. She had no problem getting on the back of my motorcycle and going for a ride in the sun, or even taking it to a soccer game in the rain for easy parking. She is a strong woman and our worlds quickly merged with our common interests.

The next few months with Isaac were amazing. I could not get enough of her time and she seemed to feel the same about me. She had three dogs, Underdog, Tank and Bear that she walked at 5:00 each morning and would not take long before I was walking them with her. I would become especially fond of Underdog, a grey and white pit bull that did not care for other dogs, but he and I got along great. I would even give Underdog a ride on my motorcycle, the same bike that Isaac and I would take to the Seattle Sounders soccer games. It was Isaac that I was visiting when I met Dr. Tauben. When I called Isaac to tell her that Tom was in ICU she immediately made arrangements to have the dogs cared for and drove to Portland and the hospital. Tom was in bad shape, the infection was getting worse quickly and I did not fully understand what was going on. I can't fathom what she thought when she saw me, but she quickly took over talking to Tom's doctors, assessing the information and helping me understand what was going on. She was also a great asset at explaining Tom's history and temperament to the attending physicians and nurses as well.

Isaac was able to spend three days with us at OHSU before she had to return to take care of her own patients. It was the first time I had an advocate that was both intellectually connected to the doctors and personally connected to me, and the relief was amazing. I felt like a great weight was lifted from me and I had complete trust that I was getting all the information to get Tom the best care as quickly as possible. Yet he was still very sick and very much fighting for his life.

After a week in ICU, Tom's health was still not improving. While I missed Isaac and her unique ability to help and create a bridge between the knowledge of the doctors and my own lack of understanding, passion, and love as a father, we were surrounded by our family and friends.

My mom was still suffering for the effects of fighting uterine cancer. The cancer had been gone for several years but the radiation had destroyed most of her digestion system. Though she could eat some things, she received most of her nutrition though a shunt that delivered what she needed directly into her blood. She dealt with a significant amount of discomfort and lethargy, however, as soon as she heard Tom was back in the hospital she was ready to leave their home and make the hour drive to OHSU.

Tom was in pain, could not eat and was growing more ill. The infection was not responding to the antibiotics. With fear and desperation in my soul I continued to reach out to everyone I could think of that might offer a solution, including Doctors Tauben and Ellenbogen. I sent them the following email.

"Tom is doing better mentally, though depressed. He was much calmer and talking normally. Physically he is still very ill. At 6'5" he weighs 127 lbs. The white counts in his blood are still elevated and the white count in the CFS is growing, the bugs are not reacting to the antibiotics. They changed the antibiotics that they are giving him (nope, I don't know what they are as I am writing this) and hoping that they will be more effective. There also is a change in his pain meds as they added Dilaudid in pill form. He ate 1/2 of an egg salad sandwich.

The neurosurgery team is still trying to keep from pulling the shunt and only replace the catheter as the infection is brought under control. It is different than the original plan for removing the shunt and putting in a ventricular drain while receiving the antibiotics. There still seems to be questions about the origin of the infection which concerns me, I would like to stop the source and not risk the problem returning.

We knew this would be a long road but it is still difficult to watch and very difficult for him to endure."

I was pleased at the response I received from Dr. Tauben. It was a message left on my voicemail that stated that though he was not Tom's attending doctor, he would be honored to be part of our journey as a friend of the family. I was greatful at his compassion and concern, and the knowledge gave us both strength.

Dr. Ellenbogen continued to follow up with the team at OHSU. He had spent ten years caring for Tom and he had taken a professional and personal interest in his wellbeing. Tom had the best professionals in the world working to get him better. However each day just dragged on.

I was afraid to leave Tom alone, and would not leave unless someone else from our family was there. Fortunately we have a great and strong family and they came every day. There was some connection to past hospital stays as we stopped at 7 Eleven on the way in and picked up a steady stream of Slurpees, but Tom was getting older and had started asking for a Starbucks white chocolate, caramel, mocha Frappuccino instead, and Starbucks was kind enough to place a store in the entry of the Children's hospital adjacent to the hospital Tom was in.

The days wore on--one week then two and three. Tom was not beating the infection and they decided that they needed to remove the valve from his brain and any foreign material where the infection could hide. The infection itself was identified as a MSRA staph infection, one that was very difficult to control.

MRSA, which stands for methicillin resistant Staphylococcus aureus, is a type of staph infection — the kind that can't be treated with first-line antibiotics. It has been referred to as the super bug that won't die, but it can, and does kill. And Tom had it rushing to his brain.

The surgery to remove the valve took a couple of hours and went well, however now Tom had the additional challenge of having an external drain coming directly from the center of his brain. The drain was attached to a bag to receive the fluid that had to be level with where his shunt left his head. If it was too high it would create pressure and additional pain. If it was too low it would drain the fluid too quickly and create a vacuum and more pain. Either issue would also cause additional concerns for damage.

I spoke to Isaac every day. She would make additional trips to Portland to visit, my family was always around, and yet I felt very much alone. Tom had been in the hospital for two weeks when my friends Clark and Terry came by to visit. Clark, a former Marine and a commander in a city police department had seen a great deal of pain and challenges. When he looked at Tom, and back at me, I saw a great deal of fear. Hope was fading and there was not much left of my son. Clark and Terry gave me hugs and prayers and left with tears in their eyes.

I watched the doctors and nurses come and go. The white blood cell counts continued to be high, and his body temperature would fluctuate from almost normal to over 103, signs that the infection still raged through his body. Tom would wake and be agitated, fighting against the calming effects of the antianxiety drugs and pain medication. He would continually press the injection button on the Dilaudid pain medication drip, before the machine regulating the maximum flow would allow the medication to be delivered.

The combined effects of the pain, fear and narcotics made Tom extremely agitated. It led me to a great deal of anger and impatience with the medical professionals. Watching my son in pain, so thin that every rib, vein, muscle, and bone was showing though his skin, caused me extreme fear, depression and sorrow. I challenged the doctors, fearing that they were not doing enough. I questioned myself, god, the universe, everything, desiring with all I had that Tom's pain would ease and he would be happy and healthy. There was so much he still had to do.

While Tom was sleeping I would doggedly climb the stairs up and down in the hospital, sometimes for hours, stopping at the fifth floor to see that he was still sleeping. It gave me something to do. I did not have to focus, just keep my feet moving as I passed doctors and nurses stairwell moving between floors.

Tom had been fighting this for more than ten years; I had been fighting with him. It needed to stop. The fear of adding more pain to my son who was already fighting a brutal battle kept me going. Someone needed to be there for him, always, and as consistently as possible. I had to believe. Ironically my greatest stress and pain was also my undeniable motivation.

Then, it broke. Twenty-four days after we had entered the emergency room, the fever broke and the white blood cell counts returned to normal, almost as if someone had thrown a switch. Two days later the doctors wheeled Tom back to surgery and replaced the shunt to drain the brain fluids through his body, this time placing it on his left side and allowing the right side to continue to heal from the trauma. He spent four more days in ICU with careful monitoring to assure that the infection would not return, and then was taken to a normal patient care room where he would spend two additional nights before I took him home.

After the surgery to replace the shunt we began short walks around the hospital. Tom was extremely weak and needed to gain strength. We had a picture taken of us outside on a small walk that went around the fourth floor, with potted flowers and a view of the city and the tram that stretches from the health center downtown by the Willamette River, up the several hundred feet to the main OHSU campus. I was so delighted that Tom was up and walking that I posted the picture of us on Facebook. To me, these were great pictures of my son healing, to others they were scary, disturbing. Looking back now I see that they looked like pictures I have seen of death camp survivors. I took them down.

The day Tom was released from the hospital he was mentally ready to go. We all felt like we could not get out of there soon enough. Though they saved his life, the trauma and memories of the pain associated with the hospital stays are overwhelming. Tom was ready to be home, see his cat, and get back to school. When we left the hospital Tom weighed just 118 pounds.

I was ready to see Isaac and get up at 5:00 AM to walk the dogs with her, but that would have to wait. Tom still had a great deal of healing to do and I needed to be with him to support him with that.

Chapter 25 - Back at Home

It was February in the Northwest and with that came long, dark nights and lots of cold rain. Tom's apartment was located along the edge of the Gresham Golf Course with a large patio door that looked out at the 14th green. The course was always green in color and from our view we could see where large ponds, small lakes really, formed in the depression along the 14th fairway.

Tom was still very weak and suffering. For the next few months I would need to stay with him and provide help with basic living needs. The apartment was warm and dry, but it was also like a small prison and the disease that had taken Tom's health was the warden that would not let us leave.

Tom had a large TV with internet connections and Netflix, so we spent our time surfing the internet and watching movies. The time passed slowly and our only release was to visit the doctor or go to the store for food. When visitors came by it was a welcome distraction, but they never stayed long.

The apartment was furnished with a second hand couch. It was a blue sectional that had some tears and stains, but it was comfortable. There was an oak coffee table that was given to Tom by our old neighbor Larry, and a lamp in the corner. For Christmas I had purchased Tom a memory foam mattress and a bed frame so that he would be a little more comfortable. In the second room I slept on the floor, on a queen sized mattress that we had gotten from my parents when they replaced it with a new set. Like the rest of Tom's place, it wasn't fancy, but it was comfortable.

Reliant or Addicted: Is There Really a Difference?

As time went by Tom did gain strength and energy. He even gained a little weight, and by the end of March he was back to 130 lbs. We made weekly trips to the doctor for checkups and pain management. It was taking more pain medication to control his head and body pain-- higher doses of Oxytocin, Norco and Dilaudid, all opiate drugs. He was also on a Percocet patch that would keep up a steady dose of the narcotic.

I was highly concerned about the amount of narcotics that Tom was taking, and expressed that to his doctors. I worried that the high doses could kill him and I was concerned about the addictions that could come with them as well. The stories I heard were always the same, Tom would likely be reliant on the narcotics for the rest of his life, but under the supervision of the doctors, he was not an addict. This was based on the theory that because he had real pain he was not addicted. The reality was that the side effects are the same, no matter what you call it. But time went by and Tom continued to get stronger and look to the future.

Tom wanted to move out of the apartment building he was in. He wanted a new place closer to the school and a new start. We started doing more together, going to movies, going on walks, visiting family, and looking for a new place to live. I started to spend more time with Isaac, and life was beginning to return to normal--as normal as it got for us.

Damn Cat

The apartment we shared was never quite clean. I am not the best housekeeper and Tom was a young, single guy with little motivation to keep his space clean. Often he would blame not cleaning, or even throwing garbage away, on not feeling well, but that became an easy excuse. The real reason was that he was a 23 year old bachelor and he just didn't care. As a 46 year old bachelor I did not have a great deal of motivation to pass the white glove test either. We did not have any dressers, though there was ample closet space. Then there was the cat, DC.

Tom's cat was large, dark with darker stripes, and rather fat.

Other than to eat and sleep, DC had one goal, to escape from the apartment. And he was quick. He was also smart. We had to be diligent about knowing where DC was any time we left the apartment and careful when we came in. As long as we acknowledged where he was at, and he knew that we knew, he would walk away from the door and all would be fine. However, if he thought we were getting ready to leave and were not paying attention to him, he would position himself so that when the door was opened he could sprint through it before we could stop him. And once he was out, it could be days before we could get him back in, and that would be because he was hungry.

We would see DC sneaking through the bushes when he got out, and about a third of the time Tom could actually catch him and bring him back in. The rest of the time it was just glimpses. One of the troubles with DC being fat was that he could go for days without eating before he came back for food. He would lose a few pounds each time he left and put it back on quickly. We fed him too much.

The Gresham Golf Course is on the edge of the city and there were a few coyotes wandering around. From time to time, we would see one out on the course, and some nights we could hear them howl. This added some stress to Tom's thoughts when DC was out. Though he seemed quick to us, he was fat, and would make a great meal for Wile E. Coyote. Tom, me and Mr. Coyote all thought it was just a matter of time. The only one that did not think so was DC. He had this.

Our other concern was the cars. The apartment complex was rather large with cars coming and going often. It was also located just off a busy road. We had seen other cats squished on the road and we did not want to see DC experience the same fate. We had seen him in the bushes, very close to the road. But then again, DC had this. He stayed away from the moving monsters.

Inside the apartment, DC was great. The large, furry beast would come to Tom when he called him and Tom had taught him to give high fives. He would do the normal kitty play with hanging balls, yarn and chasing the light of a laser pointer. And he would sit with Tom and purr as Tom stroked his soft coat. Tom and DC were friends.

A Need to Move

Tom's place was nice, a great place to live. Yet, it seemed to become depressing to him, a reminder of the pain and another failed attempt to be normal, healthy and recover. The depression was real and it was difficult to overcome. He desired a new start, a place to live that felt like progress. This place, however nice, was heavy and felt closed in. Another start, another failure, another reminder that the world was closed to him.

Tom had been through a great deal, again he had been beaten down by the disease and life, and I would do everything I could help him through. So, we started the search. We began looking for apartments that were clean, fresh, and close to Mt. Hood Community College where Tom intended to get back to his education. We found some great places and settled on Sun Point, a nice complex where he could be on the top of two floors with a small patio and a view of a large lawn and tall firs. It seemed to be a peaceful place with quiet surroundings. The quiet was important to help his head.

With the help of my parents and Glen we moved Tom into the new apartment. I found two nice dressers at the local Salvation Army and my dad brought his truck to help us move in. The dressers were very heavy but dad is tough and determined and the two of us were able to get them into the apartment and into the correct place in the bedrooms.

Tom and I found a coffee table and some matching end tables at a discount store. We ordered a sectional couch online from Walmart that arrived, but was not what we had expected. Dad stepped in again, we returned the couch and he took us to Michael's in Portland, a local furniture store, where we found a great sectional that was comfortable and long enough for Tom's 6'5" body. The couch was built in Oregon and showed us that some things are better not being imported.

The apartment had a terrific kitchen and a large, deep, Jacuzzi tub. It was less than a mile from school, a new place to live, and a chance at a new start. His new manager was kind, tried to understand Tom's situation, and was open to help Tom with what he needed. This was a place to heal.

Chapter 26 – Leaving

As Tom gained strength I spent more time back in Seattle. My mom and dad would stop by to see Tom from time to time and assure he had food. I had bought him a few cases of weight gain drinks to help him get the calories and nutrition he needed. His cousins would stop by to visit or take him out to enjoy life, and then, a girl began stopping by.

Lisa was older than Tom by several years but she seemed to really like him. She was full of energy. They told me that she was a teacher in a middle school and she was very encouraging with Tom to get back to school. She seemed to like Tom and he liked her, so life was good. I was concerned that he was getting too attached and would get his heart broken, but that was just part of life, right? I told him of my concerns but also made it clear that if she was good to him, and helped him recover, I would love her forever.

Summer in Oregon is amazing. The weather does not get too hot, and green leaves that explode with the colors of various flowers create a place of wonder. Hummingbirds zip in, out, and around the flowers and feeders that are placed near the houses and apartments. The sun brings energy as well as warmth, and it seemed to feed both of us. We went to movies, visiting my parents out in the rural spaces east of Portland, and Tom continued to heal and gain weight.

It was July when I moved back to Seattle. It was great to be back in Seattle, it was great to be back with Isaac. We spent time boating on Puget Sound, spending nights anchored off of Blake Island or in Lake Washington in Juanita Bay or just off shore from Seward Park. In August we spent Seafair Weekend tied to the log boom to watch the hydro races and air show, including the amazing Blue Angels. It was a perfect weekend for the annual event and Isaac was a great boating partner and cohost for the event. We had several people onboard and she was gracious to all of them, even the weird ones-- there were always a few of those. Life was good.

I am not sure I believe in the cliché that everything happens for a reason, but this time it seemed to work out. I was unemployed and Tom needed my time and support. However my bank accounts were depleted, and now I was back at work.

Tom and I spoke on the phone every day and he seemed to be doing well. We both had a long way to go. He needed to heal and get back to school and I needed to get into shape and get my career back on track. My financial outlook was grim, but I had enjoyed some great career success in the past, so I was not too worried. I had an amazing network of friends and associates and a track record of wild growth and strong teams--I should be back to work soon.

The first significant concern I had about Tom's new girlfriend was when she called me and asked "what are you wearing". This was an odd question for my son's girlfriend to be asking me. At first I thought it was just a silly, poorly chosen, comment but she continued to make flirtatious comments. I would visit Tom and found large quantities of women's soaps and beauty products around his house, but no Lisa.

There was also a problem with Tom's withdrawing from Mt. Hood CC and he was not able to get back into school in September, another setback. Tom was frustrated, and did not seem to be able to resolve the conflict, but was also still healing. Just nine months before he had been in ICU for a month.

He always seemed to have challenges with his finances but it seemed to be getting even worse. His bank accounts were frozen due to over drafts and lack of payments. I paid his rent and yet he was constantly out of food. His social security disability payments were not much, but he should have had ample for what he needed. It was my parents that first voiced the concern that Lisa was taking advantage of Tom and taking what little he had. I heard Tom's praise of her, and how she cared for her two nieces, and I thought that he should be able to handle himself.

Isaac and I went to Oregon for the Thanksgiving holiday. It was 2011 and Tom had been dealing with the effects of his tumor for eleven years now. Thanksgiving dinner would be at my sister's home, she had been hosting the grand meal for several consecutive years and there was a gathering of mixed family that totaled almost thirty people. The one that was missing was Tom.

Tom was still fighting severe head pain. I had been traveling back to his place in Gresham and taking him to the doctor for pain management two to three times a month. He was receiving large quantities of pain meds but they did not seem to be breaking through the heavy pain. He was also going through significant quantities of marijuana to fight the pain and nausea. He felt that the noise from the large crowd at Michelle's would make his head worse.

The meal was great-- Michelle always puts together an amazing dinner. There was the traditional turkey but there was also a stuffed prime rib roast. Someone brought sweet potatoes baked with a glaze and marshmallows. There was stuffing, hot bread, mashed potatoes and gravy, sparkling fruit juice and steelhead that Steve had caught. But all that food was only to led up to the desert bar.

As the night went, the food was consumed and people left. I made a point to stay around for a little while and help Michelle with some of the cleanup and we played some games. As it got late I fell asleep on the couch and started snoring a little. I woke startled as Michelle sprayed whipping cream from a can in my opened mouth. She and Isaac, along with whoever was left, were laughing. The lone exception was Steve who asked "Michelle, why do you do that? You know he is just going to get you back ten times worse." To which she answered "It was worth it. He is always getting me and this time he got some of his own!" I have no idea what they were talking about.

Isaac and I went in to see Tom on Friday and brought him some of the leftovers from the night's dinner. He looked fair but like he needed sleep. He was irritable and his apartment was a mess. We stopped by to see him again on the way back to Washington on Saturday, and he was still not looking real well, but after what he had been through, and was still going through with the headaches, he seemed to be doing OK.

Isaac was on call for the Christmas holiday so we spent Christmas Eve together and I went to Oregon for Christmas dinner. Tom came to the celebration at Michelle's house but did not stay long due to his head hurting. The pain was causing him to be more irritable and he would ramble about how tough it was and the amount of pain meds he was given because he was in such bad shape. He talked a lot about Lisa but did not see her either of the two holidays. I thought that a bit odd but there were still the beauty products and signs around the apartment that she had been there.

Tom was never an especially clean person but his habits were getting worse. His apartment was filled with filled trash bags. He had been smoking cigarettes and the manager of the complex complained that he was tossing the butts on the stairs and around the outside walkway. There were butts outside, but Tom swore that it was the neighbors that were making the mess.

Over the next few weeks I received calls from the property manager complaining about Tom, people coming and going at odd hours, his girlfriend's attitude and various problems. He neighbors were complaining. At the same time Tom complained about the manager, called her a bitch, and said that she was harassing him. She did not like his girlfriend.

One evening in February I received a call from Tom telling me he needed some extra money because Lisa had parked in the wrong spot and the apartment manager had her car towed. He said it was his responsibility and he needed to come up with the money, $350, to get her car out. He wanted me to wire the money immediately. I declined, and he became very stressed.

A few days later I received a call from Lisa. She told me Tom was out of control and something needed to be done. He needed help. I asked her what she meant and she talked about him being angry, unreasonable, and not taking care of himself. She also talked about the money she had to come up with to get her car back from being towed. The call was odd and I had the strong impression that she wanted me to send her money for the car bill. She reiterated that Tom owed her several hundred dollars. I suggested that she stop seeing him then. This was the first of several calls, most of which I just let go to voice mail.

The complaints increased from the apartment manager and I returned to Oregon to see what was going on with Tom and see if I could help him. When I walked into his apartment I noticed that his large screen TV was gone. There was also a large hole in the wall of his hall way and some of the cabinets in the kitchen were broken. There were still women's beauty products around the house, Lisa was still around.

I asked Tom about Lisa and what was going on. He told me how much he loved her and what a great person she was. It was Lisa that was taking him to the doctors now and making sure he took care of himself. The stories of how great she was to him, and how caring she was to her two nieces, did not make sense to me, with the calls she made to me complaining about Tom. I was slow, did not want to believe what I was seeing, but it was becoming evident that Tom had lost control of his medications and had become an addict. Tom was alone, not feeling well on a cold night in January when he received the phone call. It was a man asking if Lisa was with him. He said no, and the man began to push about where she might be. Tom asked who it was and he said "I am her husband." He did not want to believe it but he knew that she was. All the stories and time apart, he knew it was odd.

His head was already hurting and he was feeling the usual nausea that came along with the opiates. He wanted to throw up, to cry, to yell, and to hit something. He did all three. Each time he went to the doctor he received prescriptions for hundreds of pills, quantities that would kill most people that had not developed the tolerance that he had. And she had been helping him. Lisa brought people that would buy Tom's pills, and for a fraction of the cost they could buy meth that helped his headaches. Tom had become a different person, sad, mean, and centered only on Lisa, drugs and himself. When Lisa finally showed up she told him that she and her husband had an open relationship and that she was afraid to tell Tom because he might leave her. She also admitted that the kids she had told Tom were her nieces, where in fact her daughters. She told him how much she loved, told him that she was filing for divorce so they could be together. He loved her. She was all he had, and he would do anything for her, everything for her, and he did.

By March, Tom had sold all his furniture. He claimed that it had been stolen. He was also given a final eviction notice. He was sleeping with friends at times and outside at others. Isaac and I had gone down to see him and we had to meet at a restaurant, he said he was sleeping outside. I asked him to come back to Seattle with me but he would not. He was still trying to work out things with Lisa and had to stay in Oregon. It made me sick to see him this way, but I did not know what else to do, so I went home to Seattle. I knew he was buying and selling drugs and that it had cost him everything. By this point it had cost me almost all I had as well. I paid for his apartments, furniture, a great deal of his food and medicines and covered that thousands of dollars in overdraft fees. In retrospect, I realized that I had been part of the problem, enabling him to finance his fall into a dark hole. I was depressed as well.

Isaac was young, an accomplished doctor, and she was ready to start a family. I had been through hell with Tom's health, my divorce, and my own health. I had decided that there was no way I was going to start a new family. I can still remember the warm spring day that she told me she could no longer be my lover. Things were falling apart in my life. I was alone in Seattle, I would still talk to Tom every couple of days when he would answer his phone. He still had a cell phone. I continued to pay that bill so I could reach him.

I met Barb on a nice day for lunch at my favorite Italian place in Bellevue. She worked for Microsoft and my office was close by. She was medium height with blonde hair and big blue eyes. She had a great smile, smart and talked about her two young kids, playing guitar and her job as a program manager. We had a great meal but she seemed to be in a different world and not especially interested in getting together again. We shook hands and said goodbye.

Two days later Barb called and asked me to lunch. We talked about meeting at Microsoft and then agreed to meet at a Thai restaurant between our offices. We had another nice conversation that was friendly. At the end of our meal I walked her back to her car and gave her a hug.

We talked about getting together again and going out on the boat for the weekend. My life was a mess and she had a lot going on, so I sent her the story from Mary Swift and the Seattle PI--it was an easy way to say that I had MS and a son that had high needs. I don't know what went through her mind when she read the article, in the past it would end relationships quickly, but she still wanted to spend a day on the lake with me. It would be sometime later that I learned that she had already seen the article, even before we met the first time. She was a Microsoft technology geek and she had found everything about me that had been recorded and published online.

Out on the lake we talked about life, a great deal about Tom and his struggles, and living with MS. She spoke about being a single mom, what she had been through after her divorce, and going back to working at Microsoft to support her family. Why she decided she wanted to continue going out with me I don't know, but I am grateful.

A week after I met Barb, the president of the company I was working for flew up unannounced and fired me. Six months earlier I had taken over the Seattle operations of the small magazine that had been losing money for over a year. We had grown the revenues by 70% and were close to a breakeven point but it was not good enough. Just a few weeks later they closed the Seattle office and stopped circulation in the Northwest completely. It was June, I was out of work, my son was out of control and hurting and I was depressed and lost.

Chapter 27 - Hitting Rock Bottom

I made several trips back to Oregon to see Tom and do what I could to help him in June. I stayed with my parents, who were very concerned. Tom had stayed with them for a couple of days but quickly began fighting with my father. He could not stay there. My mom was already weak from her long battle from the effects of cancer, and the extra stress was enormous. Tom was choosing to be homeless.

It was close to the middle of July when Tom finally decided to come back to Seattle with me and stay on the boat. He immediately called the doctors here and talked his way into more massive amounts of opiates. His legs hurt and he was having trouble walking. He was very angry and I looked for ways to help him find reasons to smile. He did have some time where he would be able to control himself but it was tough. Barb really seemed to love Tom. She was always happy and he began to call her Mary Poppins, we both did. She was all mom, had kids of her own, and hurt for us when we hurt, and continued to give us smiles.

At the end of July Tom went to visit a friend in Tacoma. I received that call in the late evening from his friend that I needed to come pick him up. They were concerned that he had overdosed. I drove as quickly as I could and found Tom awake and jabbering. They told me that some other kids had come over and brought Tom some drugs, though they were not sure what. Tom had gone in the bathroom and taken out everything from every cabinet. Then he passed out in the tub, which was when they called.

Tom was wobbling, almost could not walk. In the car on the way back to Seattle he was going in and out of consciousness. I sent a texts to Isaac and Mary asking for advice. They both told me to get him to the hospital and Isaac told me she would meet me at Harborview. When I pulled up Tom became excessively angry, almost violent. Isaac was there waiting for us, she was stressed. I called for her help and she came, it was a great deal to ask and likely the last time I would see her, but I would do anything to find help for Tom. He told them he had not taken anything, had not told me he would kill himself. They did take him in to watch for suicidal behavior. The doctor caring for him told me he had tested positive for cocaine and meth.

Hair Cut

"Damn, I need a haircut." Tom was irritated and frustrated. He had spent the money he had, on who knows what, and he did not have any money to take care of himself. His head had been hurting, life just generally sucked. It had been so long, his hair was long and shaggy, and he could not even get a haircut.

He wasn't happy with me. He was not happy with anyone. The pain pills and other drugs he had turned to were not providing much relief. In fact, his legs were hurting more, and he needed a damn haircut!

Finally, he decided he would do what whatever it would take to cut his hair, even do it himself. His ataxia was making him shake more, he was unstable, very much like a drunk person--this would be interesting.

Just about that time, our friend Betty came over to see how Tom was doing. She had just come from having a beer at a local pub. We started talking and sharing shots of tequila. As we listened to Tom tell stories we had several shots of tequila. Pretty soon she was tipsy. It was about then that she and Tom decided it would be a good idea for her to give Tom a haircut. I had a very difficult time not laughing.

Drunken girl giving a haircut to a stoned guy that can't sit still--what could go wrong? Despite the massive amounts of opiates Tom had taken, his head was still tender, and every time Betty hit his skin with the metal of the cutters he would send out a shriek or tirade of profanity.

When it was done I was taking pictures on my smart phone and sending them off to a few select friends. I called my mom. As I explained what was happening to my mom, the kind woman that loves Tom with every fiber of her heart broke out laughing.

Life gives you lessons, like this one: do not let a drink girl cut your hair, especially when you are stoned as well.

Tom left the boat and continued his downslide. He was angry, yelling, and almost unable to walk. A few days earlier he had cleaned everything on the boat to a sparkling shine. Hours later he was looking for his pills, could not find them ,and tore the boat apart looking for them, for one, for anything. He was so desperate he pulled the vacuum and vacuum bag apart to see if anything has been sucked up while he was cleaning.

He was upset and had put a large amount of my clothes into the washing machine at the end of the dock and filled it with bleach, various cleaners he could find, and left. He would not talk to me, other than to swear and call me names, and then went to sleep on a small hill in Seattle with other homeless people.

While Tom was there other men came to take his drugs, any money he might have, or just to kick him. The police would come by and tell him he could not stay there. He had no friends, no one would answer his calls, and eventually his phone was stolen.

I did not know what to do. I reached out to my friends that had been around drug addictions and they told me that there was nothing I could do until Tom decided to help himself. I called the King County addiction hotline and they told me the same thing. I looked for ways to get him committed to a treatment center, but laws in Washington do not allow for that.

I finally reached the Executive Director for the King County Addiction Center and she told me there was nothing I could do. She had lost her husband to drugs and her son had become an addict. She lost track of him for several years before he had returned after he had cleaned up. All that time she waited for a call to say that he had overdosed. The advice I was given by multiple professionals was to cut off contact with Tom. He had to decide to commit himself to an addiction center and if I allowed him to return, give him money, or even feed him, I was enabling him and his addiction.

On the day that I had spoken to the ED for King County Addiction, I also received a call from my friend Richard Werlien. I had met Werlien at his house when another friend had invited me over for a poker game. After the game Werlien invited me to return and we quickly became friends, attending concerts, sporting events and other activities. Werlien had his own business that is extremely busy in the summer and almost nonexistent in the winter. He is an outspoken, at times crass, an ex-marine with a strong and loud personality. I have no doubt that Werlien can be judgmental, but he is also a loyal friend without question and will not hesitate to do what he believes is the right thing.

Rich called, probably to ask be about poker and I told him the advice I had been give about Tom. His immediate response, that confirmed what I was feeling, was "FUCK THAT! You do what you have to do to get Tom healthy and off that shit." He sounded thoroughly pissed off. His anger at the situation, the advice I was given, the tone I had that there was nothing I could do, gave me a much needed shock to my system. Somebody had to be in Tom's corner and reach out to him, no matter what. He might go down, but if that happened we were going down together.

Chapter 28 - Won't Let Tom Go Again

I have always blamed Tom's death on drugs, but in reality he was shot by a reserve police officer as he was running from a vacant house that he and another boy had broken into. I heard that the officers had been drinking and there were many questions surrounding that night. It was dark, storming, raining hard that night in a rural area east of Portland, Oregon. I was not there. I should have been. Tom and I did everything together. When I think back to the time that I learned of his death, that day comes back as if it were just a few hours ago.

I was 16, shopping at Sharon's Pantry, the only real grocery store in Sandy, Oregon at the time. The night before it had rained like crazy but today the sun had broken out. I was back by the dairy products when our school bus driver saw me and came to say how sorry she was about my friend. I had no idea what, or who, she was talking about. Then she said his name, and how she always really liked Tom and me.

I still did not understand what was going on. I made my purchase and got in the car to drive home. On the radio the song was playing, Seasons in the Sun. That song was playing a lot at that time, still popular though it had been released some years before. I remember the lyrics, "Goodbye my friend, it's hard to die." Then the news came on about a teenager being shot and killed in Sandy. When I got home my parents were stressed and wanted to talk with me. They told me that Tom had been shot the night before and had died.

Tom and I had met when their family moved to the area where my family and I lived. Tom and his sister Anne were a year apart in age but they both were in the eighth grade with me at Bull Run, a small school teaching grades one through eight, two grades per class, with 78 kids in the entire school. We became friends almost immediately and hardly separated.

Tom and I had horses and rode them everywhere. As soon as school was out we got to the horses, and most of the time Anne was with us. Our houses were two miles apart and we would walk, or ride, between the houses daily.

Before I met Tom I was pretty much an introvert, a loner. I did not have real friends at school and most of my time was spent in front of the TV. Tom was popular and energetic with a large, shit eating grin. Everyone seemed to like him. He was quick witted and could talk his way, our way, out of most trouble. My friendship with Tom dramatically changed my life.

When we were in grade school we rode horses, played sports, and caused as much trouble as possible on horseback. There was a lake with a park between our houses, Lake Roslyn. We fished along the lake and played in the park. The rules forbade us from riding our horses in the park so we found trails and ways to get into the park that were not monitored by the ranger. That included riding our horses into the lake and swimming them to the park. If we were up early, we would ride through the park and appropriate any lunch boxes or coolers that fishermen had left on the picnic tables.

As we got older we attended school at Sandy High, where we found an interest in girls. I always had a crush on Anne. Sometimes it was obvious, sometimes I was able to keep it to myself. Tom was popular and had friends, and so I had friends. I remember that one day a cute girl, Christy, started talking to me in class. She and her friends were great and fun for a few days. Then Tom told her that I had a crush on her. A few days later she was distant and cold. Tom got upset with her for some reason and told her we thought she was a bitch. So went my high school love life. Tom included me in everything and we had upgraded from swiping lunch boxes to going for joy rides in my parents car or the occasional car parked around the lake.

When we borrowed a car from around the lake, we would have found an extra key, usually in the glove box or under the floor mat of an unlocked car. We would drive it around for a bit and then park it a ways from where we found it. We almost got in wrecks a couple of times, but we managed to miss them, miss the police, and not do any real damage.

Tom included me in everything. That started to change when I met a cute girl at church--we were both Mormon and Tom was Catholic. Tom went to church with me once or twice but was given grief about being Catholic, so he stopped, but there were the cute girls, so I kept going. I started drifting from my friend.

I knew Tom had smoked pot. We were together when one of his friends offered us a joint and he declined, became upset and let everyone know that I did not smoke and it was not OK to ask me. Tom was always a true friend and cared about who I was. I knew he had taken pills a couple of times, but it did not seem like a big deal.

To this day I feel guilty for not being with Tom that night. I know it is cliché, but if we had been together, that night would have been different. I had gone out with my church friends to a dance and left Tom. I had walked away from the friend that had included me in everything. Part of my reasoning at the time was because Tom was smoking pot and I did not want to be part of that. The real reason, I was worried about myself.

In my mind Tom was probably high that night. I have no real reason to think that, but it has given me a reason for all these years to blame his death on drugs, an evil part of this world, and I was not there. Tom was my best friend, had been for years. I carried his casket with his brothers and I still grieve today. I named my son after him. I left my friend to deal with tough challenges on his own and I lost him. I am not going to walk away from my son.

Chapter 29 - Then Tom Came Back

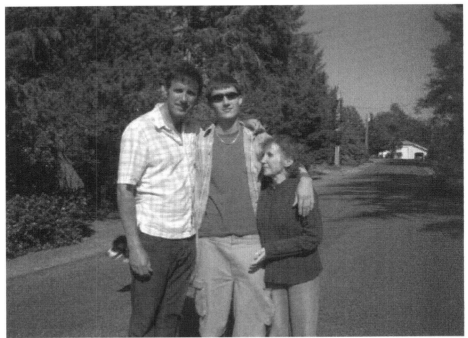

Tom, his Grandma Charlotte and me during his first month of recovery. We were visiting Long Beach, Washington.

Rich's words gave me the boost I needed and I continued to do what I could to see Tom, give him food and let him know that I was there for him. Tom came back to the boat and asked if he could have something to eat, and maybe a place to sleep. I answered yes, but he would have to meet a friend of mine and spend a day with him.

Kellee is an amazing friend. She is a professor at Seattle Pacific University and connected with the world. She has piercing blue eyes that seem to look though you and communicate with your soul. We became friends though her partner Suzanne, the Chair of the Puget Sound Leadership Council while I worked with the American Cancer Society. They both had become my friends and Kellee was out to help me find a job. Kellee introduced me to Peter, who had connections to a nonprofit center that dealt with autism. I went to meet Peter at his day job, the Matt Tabor Center, a place for homeless drug addicts.

Peter and I went to lunch and talked about the center and Tom. He is an amazing and caring guy and said he would like to meet Tom and would make sure he got introduced and what he needed if he chose to come in. The timing was incredible. Peter told me he believed things happen for a reason.

I took Tom to meet Peter and he spent two days at the center, nights he would come back to the boat. At the end of two days, he told me he was done, he was going to quit taking all drugs. He was sincere. Tom was addicted to a combination of opiates and Benzodiazepines. Withdrawal from Benzos can be fatal, so on August 9, 2012, we checked Tom into Swedish Medical Center in Ballard for three days where they monitored him. He refused to take any methadone or other drugs to help with the addictions, being aware that they come with addictions and side effects of their own. On the third day, Tom moved back on the boat to stay with me.

The next few months were exceptionally brutal to watch. The withdrawals for the drugs Tom had been taking can last for year, but the first months are the worst. His head hurt, his body ached. Every cell in his body seemed as if it wanted to explode. He would be cold and then break into a burning sweat. For what seemed to be no reason at all he would become extremely angry, and then cry. He continued to smoke cigarettes but nothing else.

The company I was working for had closed its offices in Washington. Tom needed around the clock care so I focused on helping him. For the next year we lived on savings and some small consulting jobs I picked up from time to time.

Tom would spend as much of the time as possible in his room. He would read or use his computer when he could. We would go to the store most days just to have something to do. At nights when he was sleeping he would let out screams, or sob, something that still haunts us today.

When Tom was sleeping, as I had done so many times before, I would listen through his door to hear if he was breathing. When I wasn't sure, I would slightly open the door and if I needed, I would call his name until he grunted "huh."

WILLIE!

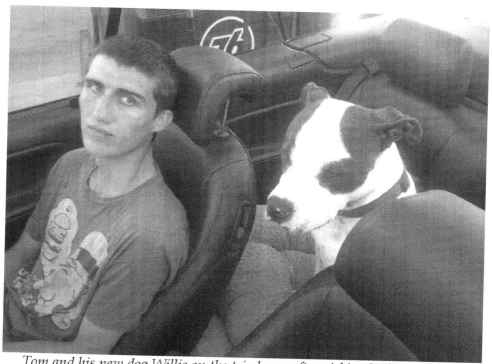

Tom and his new dog Willie on the trip home after picking Willie up from the humane society in Port Orchard, Washington.

Tom needed a friend, something to focus on. I needed a friend, too, so we found Willie. Willie is a large black and white dog we found at the Port Townsend Humane society. He was just a year old, with lots of energy. His is one big muscle formed into a puppy. Searching the internet we decided that he most closely resembles an American Bull Dog. He also looks a lot like a big Pit Bull.

Willie is full of love without a hint of aggression. He has separation issues and has chewed most of the things in the boat when left behind, but when we go to sleep he wants nothing more than to cuddle up. Barb was concerned about him being aggressive around her small kids. His is a pig and highly food motivated, but is extremely gentle, letting her six year old daughter Emily get down with him in his food dish, take his food out and feed it to him by hand. My mother, a very soft spoken, conservative woman, that everyone loves, and never swears, surprised us all when she said "he is just a big pussy." My dad almost fell over as he said "Charlotte, we have been married over fifty years and I have never heard you use that term!"

There is a lot to read about service animals and the emotional support pets can give. With Willie and Tom, every bit of it is true. Willie is large, strong, and happy and wants to play. Tom has a friend to play with, love, and receive love from. He tells Willie every day "nobody likes you", as he gives him treats and plays with him on the boat. The bond between the two of them is immense. Willie has been a great companion for me too. I am calmer with him, more consistent, and he reacts well to that. He will obey me at times when he ignores Tom, but his love and loyalty to both of us is tangible. He has been a wonder at helping Tom stay off drugs and gives him focus when I am not around.

Willie is not perfect, but I think he may be perfect for us. None of us have much grace or balance, a challenge for us living on a boat, and added to that, Willie is one big muscle, no fat, and sinks without a doggie lifejacket. He has about the same level of concentration as Tom and I have, and all of these factors have contributed to him falling off the dock and into the lake, **THREE TIMES IN ONE WINTER!**

For Christmas of 1012, Tom gave me an incredible gift. He quit smoking. Again, he quit "cold turkey". He tells me that at times it is harder than the drugs. His resolve is amazing and I have my son back.

In February, Barb bought a new car. She chose a minivan, really a matchbox van from Mazda. In reality it is a great car for her and her two kids. She gave her old car, a 2007, Saturn Vue, to Tom. The Vue has some rough wear, a few bumps and scars, and it keeps going. It fits in well with our lives.

A month ago Tom had a tooth that developed an abscess and required a root canal. The depth was unusual and the first dentist had to send him to a specialist. The process is painful, and combined with the chronic head pain from his traumatic brain surgeries, it is even more so for Tom. The dentist gave him Vicodin for the pain, and he gave me the pills. "Dad, I really want to get through this without pills, I don't want to become addicted again." And he did. It has been nine months since he has had a narcotic or drink of alcohol, and four months since he has had a cigarette. He is one tough young man.

"You know dad, there is something I learned about myself. I can do anything if I think it needs to be done--I just do it." Tom was talking to me as we walked along Westlake Avenue in Seattle on his way to the dentist. "I decided to give up the drugs and I did. I just did it. I quit smoking and I am back in school. The other day the neighbor's boat died and was bumping into other boats and I jumped in to get the rope from them and pull it to the other side, and that water was fucking cold." We kept walking, and as I listened to him, Willie pulled to the side to sniff something. "I think I got my toughness from you, we both just do what needs to be done. You are going to get your career and job straightened out, just because it needs to be done. We don't have to worry."

Chapter 30 – Introductions

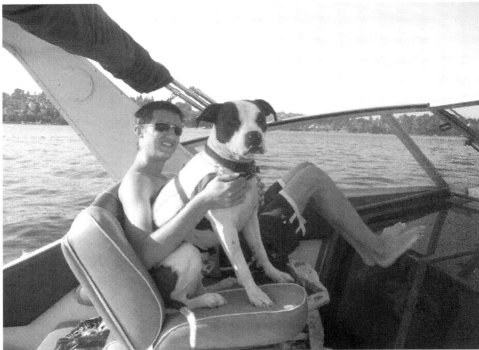

Tom and his dog Willie out on the Boat in Lake Washington. Willie is wearing a life jacket because we learned he will jump in the water but he can't swim, he sinks.

Let me introduce you to Tom. He is still a slob. Every day he fights pain and challenges that resulted from the disease and treatments. Every day is a challenge to get up and take control of the day. He loves kids and they love him. He will give you all he has if he thinks you need it. He is generous to a fault. He has traveled through hell and beaten back the fires and still can conjure a smile that will brighten a room. He can sympathize and empathize with those in pain. He has a goal to not only be self-sustaining, but to work with special needs kids and make this world a better place. At 6'5" and 150 lbs., I still call him a straw, he is too skinny to be a stick. He can talk to anybody and everybody without fear, for he has faced both God and Satan.

Tom and I play poker once a month with David Allen and our group of friends. Our old neighbor Scott is there, with our close friends Stickland, Werlien and Lancaster. These are just a few of the people that have kept us afloat through the years. From time to time we play cards at Werlien's. From time to time Tom wins. He is smart, driven, and a joy to be around. When we play, we are with friends that have seen us at our lowest and our highest. They still invite us back, give us hugs, and then we try to take their money. Tom is one tough young man with an incredible, though old, spirit and soul. He has the strength and heart I always wish I had. He is the son I always knew I had, my closest friend. It has been my deepest fear that I will write the end to this story. There have been times that I lost hope, and yet somehow Tom finds the strength to keep the story going. So if you want to know the end of this story you will have to wait. Wait and ask Tom.

38150369R00112

Made in the USA
Charleston, SC
29 January 2015